The Survival Medical Handbook & Long Term Disaster Preparedness Guide

2 IN 1 COMPILATION

MODERN DAY PREPPERS SECRETS TO SURVIVE ANY CRISIS WHEN HELP IS NOT ON THE WAY

Small Footprint Press

THIS COLLECTION INCLUDES THE FOLLOWING BOOKS:

The Survival Medical Handbook

The Worst-Case Survival Book For Disaster Preparedness

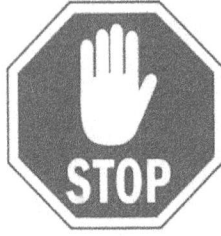

BEFORE YOU START READING, DOWNLOAD YOUR FREE BONUSES!

Scan the QR-code & Access
all the Resources for FREE!

SCAN ME

https://dl.bookfunnel.com/h8hzy33mn7

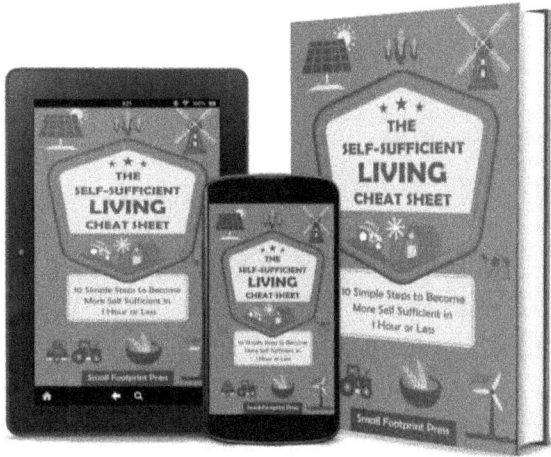

The Self-Sufficient Living Cheat Sheet

10 Simple Steps to Become More Self-Sufficient in 1 Hour or Less

How to restore balance to the environment around you... even if you live in a tiny apartment in the city.

Discover:

- **How to increase your income** by selling "useless" household items

- The environmentally friendly way to replace your car — invest in THIS special vehicle to **eliminate your carbon footprint**

- The secret ingredient to **turning your backyard into a thriving garden**

- 17+ different types of food scraps and 'waste' that you can use to feed your garden

- How to drastically **cut down on food waste** without eating less

- 4 natural products you can use to make your own eco-friendly cleaning supplies

- The simple alternative to 'consumerism' — the age-old method for **getting what you need without paying money for it**

- The 9 fundamental items you need to create a self-sufficient first-aid kit

- One of the top skills that most people are afraid of learning — and how you can master it effortlessly

- 3 essential tips for **gaining financial independence**

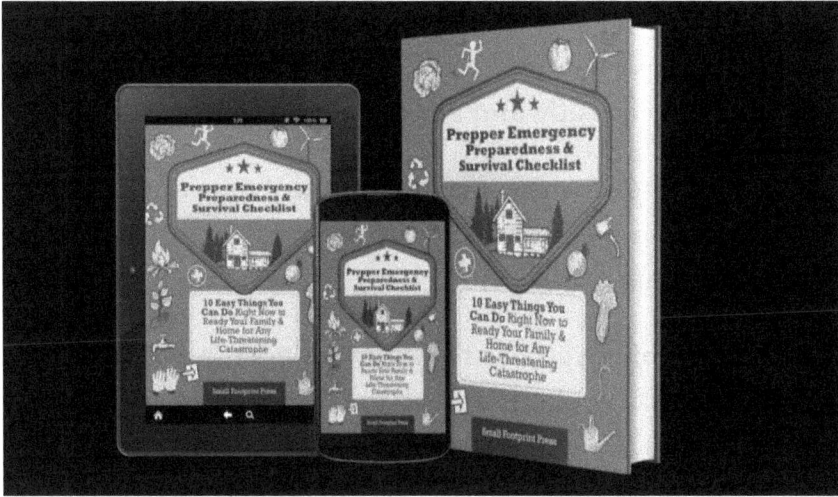

The Prepper Emergency Preparedness & Survival Checklist:

10 Easy Things You Can Do Right Now to Ready Your Family & Home for Any Life-Threatening Catastrophe

Natural disasters demolish everything in their path, but your peace of mind and sense of safety don't have to be among them. Here's what you need to know...

- Why having an emergency plan in place is so crucial and how it will help to keep your family safe

- How to stockpile emergency supplies intelligently and why you shouldn't overdo it

- How to store and conserve water so that you know you'll have enough to last you through the crisis

- A powerful 3-step guide to ensuring financial preparedness, no matter what happens

- A step-by-step guide to maximizing your storage space, so you and your family can have exactly what you need ready and available at all times

- Why knowing the hazards of your home ahead of time could save a life and how to steer clear of these in case of an emergency

- Everything you need to know for creating a successful evacuation plan, should the worst happen and you need to flee safely

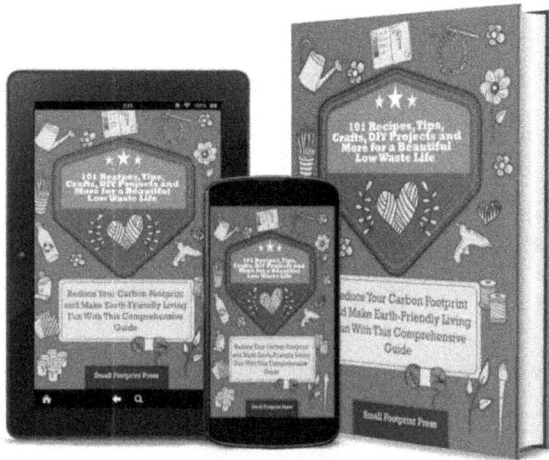

101 Recipes, Tips, Crafts, DIY Projects and More for a Beautiful Low Waste Life

Reduce Your Carbon Footprint and Make Earth-Friendly Living Fun With This Comprehensive Guide

Practical, easy ways to improve your personal health and habits while contributing to a brighter future for yourself and the planet

Discover:

- **Simple customizable recipes for creating your own food, home garden, and skincare products**

- The tools you need for each project to successfully achieve sustainable living

- Step-by-step instructions for life-enhancing skills from preserving food to raising your own animals and forging for wild berries

- **Realistic life changes that reduce your carbon-footprint while saving you money**

- Sustainable crafts that don't require any previous knowledge or expertise

- Self-care that extends beyond the individual and positively impacts the environment

- **Essential tips on how to take back control of your life -- become self-sustained and independent**

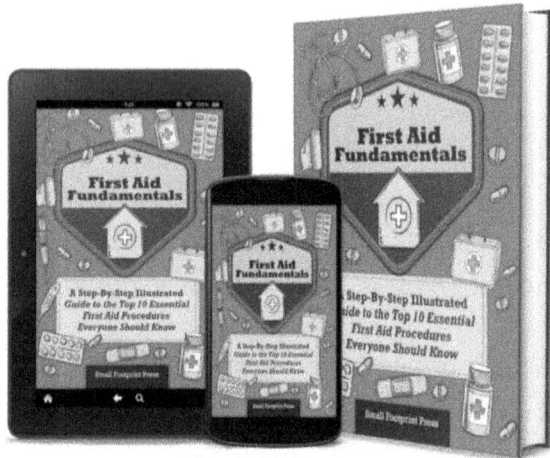

First Aid Fundamentals

A Step-By-Step Illustrated Guide to the Top 10 Essential First Aid Procedures Everyone Should Know

Discover:

- **What you should do to keep this type of animal attack from turning into a fatal allergic reaction**

- Why sprains are more than just minor injuries, and how you can keep them from getting worse

- **How to make the best use of your environment in critical situations**

- The difference between second- and third-degree burns, and what you should do when either one happens

- Why treating a burn with ice can actually cause more damage to your skin

- When to use heat to treat an injury, and when you should use something cold

- **How to determine the severity of frostbite**, and what you should do in specific cases

- Why knowing this popular disco song could help you save a life

- The key first aid skill that everyone should know — **make sure you learn THIS technique the right way**

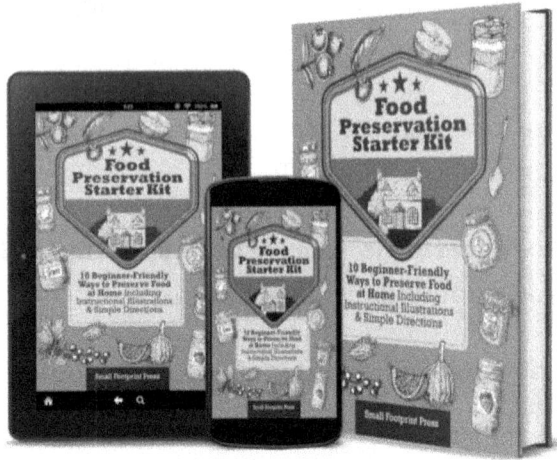

Food Preservation Starter Kit

10 Beginner-Friendly Ways to Preserve Food at Home | Including Instructional Illustrations and Simple Directions

Grocery store prices are skyrocketing! It's time for a self-sustaining lifestyle.

Discover:

- **10 incredibly effective and easy ways to preserve your food for a self-sustaining lifestyle**

- The art of canning and the many different ways you can preserve food efficiently without any prior experience

- A glorious trip down memory lane to learn the historical methods of preservation passed down from one generation to the next

- **How to make your own pickled goods**: enjoy the tanginess straight from your kitchen

- Detailed illustrations and directions so you won't feel lost in the preservation process

- The health benefits of dehydrating your food and how fermentation can be **the key to a self-sufficient life**

- **The secrets to living a processed-free life** and saving Mother Earth all at the same time

Download all your resources by scanning the QR-Code below:

SCAN ME

https://dl.bookfunnel.com/h8hzy33mn7

CONTENTS

THE SURVIVAL MEDICAL HANDBOOK

INTRODUCTION

"Care shouldn't start in the emergency room,"

—*James Douglas.*

We agree with James Douglas when it comes to first aid and preparing for emergencies. A little foresight, the right knowledge, and the determination to help another can often prevent major emergencies and even save a life.

We don't mean to candy-coat the grit needed to do this, nor to downplay your anxiety at the thought of dealing with medical emergencies and other injuries. However, we at Small Footprint Press believe that, of the obstacles preventing you from helping another in distress, the overwhelming panic you might feel is the greatest. We further believe that this panic stems from not knowing the right steps to help a person in distress, along with the fear that you may worsen the situation instead of helping. We understand this as we have been there ourselves; but we have also discovered that familiarity with standard basic first aid empowers you to act for the best outcome with the least anguish to all concerned.

To that end, we've compiled this step-by-step guide outlining common situations requiring first aid, how to prepare to administer first aid, how to identify what steps are needed, and how to preserve life until professional help can reach you. We've included how to prepare for medical emergencies before they occur, and what items you should have on hand for basic first aid and common minor emergencies at home, work, or while traveling.

Our aim is not to overwhelm, but to present you with steps you can take to prepare for medical emergencies, along with techniques that are simple to do and effective in preserving life or reducing visits to hospital emergency rooms.

We don't expect to turn you into a medical professional. Instead, we hope to provide you with the knowledge to assist a person in distress or a life-threatening situation until the paramedics or other first responders arrive.

As times change and natural and civic emergencies grow steadily, you may need to prepare to preserve life and monitor someone who is ill for a longer than expected period as rescue professionals may not always reach you as soon as you hope. For this reason, we've extended our "be prepared and let's prevent it" philosophy toward first aid as well. At the end of the book, you'll find some alternative remedies and treatments that can be easily made or done at home to preserve life and promote recovery.

About Small Footprint Press

"Accelerating Sustainable Survival for the Individual and our Planet"

"Prepping to survive a global catastrophe goes hand-in-hand with stopping the destruction of our planet by living sustainably!" Small Footprint Press Company Values.

While we aren't Doomers who believe the worst is inevitable sooner rather than later, nor are we of the belief that the end of the world is arriving, we do believe in being prepared for the worst while living your best life each day. For this reason, we work toward promoting and encouraging sustainable, prepared living as an individual. Yes, many would call us Preppers, while an equal number would call us like-minded individuals. Did you know that in 2021 over 45 percent of Americans, both men and women, invested towards prepping for worst-case scenarios? (Laycock & Choi, 2021) We're not just talking about stockpiling food and toilet paper, but also equipment and taking instructional courses.

We hope that this guide will be one that you choose to add to your preparedness, not just for natural disasters or service collapses, but also for those recreational and everyday situations that suddenly turn into emergencies through unforeseen circumstances or environmental factors such as severe storms and isolated locations. In doing so, we thank you for helping to preserve and sustain life while promoting recovery—extending your first aid mindset to not just people in distress, but to the world at large too.

Disclaimer

This book seeks to educate and present first aid techniques and procedures in an easy-to-understand way using the most up-to-date information. In doing so, we take no responsibility for the outcomes of your performance of the techniques and procedures, whether those outcomes are good or bad. We offer you this knowledge in good faith and understanding that this information will be used only when required and with good intentions.

While we mention certain brand name medications, our intention is not to promote those products, merely to inform you of the brand names we feel most people would be familiar with and which are easily obtainable. Please use the medications of the distressed person if those are known, and your medications of choice to stock your personal first aid kits.

Regarding the natural remedies and medicinal recipes in this book, please read this disclaimer at the chapter beginning, and all warnings and cautions for all remedies.

How to Use this Book

Use the first and last chapters, You Cannot Be Prepared Enough and Alternative Medicines for Emergencies to prepare yourself mentally, gather your first aid items and first aid kits, as well as your medical emergency kits for members of your family.

Use the second chapter, Good-to-Learn Techniques, to familiarize yourself with the most often used and effective techniques for treating a variety of situations. We recommend reading through this chapter more than once, and to regularly refresh your memory by reading it at the beginning of summer and the middle of winter just before most seasonal injuries usually occur.

Read through the third, fourth, and fifth chapters, Mild Emergencies, Serious Emergencies, and Responding to Emergencies Related to Permanent Conditions. This will raise your awareness of some of the symptoms and ways to respond to a range of emergencies. If you encounter an emergency and have this guide available, you can quickly go through the steps or look at symptoms again. If there's no time to access this guide, that's okay, you'll have your familiarity with the major techniques that could still save a life.

We thank you in advance for the good you're about to send out at times when it is truly needed. Now, let's get you on the path to preserving life!

Chapter 1:

You Cannot Be Ready Enough

You can't be ready enough, that's true, but you can be prepared to the best of your ability. While our environment and services degrade and disasters become more frequent, we cannot afford complacency or to rely on the expectation that medical help will always be on hand or reach us in a timely manner. It falls more and more on us to take up the slack for our own good and that of our fellow beings.

When situations arise where there is no available medical help or rescue, you will need to be prepared to offer first aid. Before we tackle situations and techniques, we will look at how you can be prepared to meet emergencies before they occur.

When to Call an Emergency Number

When to call an emergency number seems like a silly question, but there are times when you *shouldn't* call an emergency number, or times when even though you've called for help, it may not reach you and the person in distress in time. Imagine, for example, there's been a tornado, your house is in ruins, and your elderly parent has a head injury that is bleeding profusely. Naturally, you need to call emergency services, but in the interminable time it takes them to clear a path to your house and reach you and your

7

parent, it's up to you to offer first aid and keep your parent lucid.

You're not a doctor no matter your level of first aid knowledge (unless, of course, you hold a medical doctor's degree) and no-one expects you to perform surgery or long-term treatment. The advice we offer is to help you prepare as much as you can in the event no medical care is immediately available.

Remember, when there's no-one else to offer medical help, you should follow the appropriate steps described for each emergency and seek help as fast as possible.

In the event medical assistance is available, but you are unsure what constitutes an urgent medical situation, you will want to check the following list.

What Constitutes an Emergency Situation

- The person is in a life-threatening condition. For example, they are experiencing severe bleeding that won't stop, severe allergic reaction, a heart attack, severe abdominal pain or continuous vomiting, or it's a case of poisoning or a motor accident.

- The person's condition is deteriorating fast and you believe their condition could become life-threatening en route to the hospital.

- Relocating or shifting the person into a new position may cause further injury. For example, they have a neck or spine injury or have been in a severe accident.

- A paramedic's skills and equipment are required to treat or stabilize the person.

- Transportation to the hospital may be delayed because of your location, weather, or traffic conditions.

The Three Cs of Emergency

To help you remember how to respond to an emergency while keeping yourself and others safe as your assist, we have The Three Cs and The Three Ps of first aid. These Cs and Ps also ensure you do not panic and that you approach the situation as safely as possible.

First do the three Cs. Check, Call, Care.

Check

Check for dangers in the environment and in the area around the person, for example if a house is on fire, or they are at the edge of a storm torrent. If there is a clear or imminent danger, you may require help in assisting further, or you may need to make a plan to reach the person safely. Being aware of dangers and prudently approaching the emergency prevents further emergencies and ensures more effective and efficient courses of action for you and the responding medics.

This also ensures less harm is done to the injured person and to others in the area. The worst thing to do is to rush into a situation without being aware of further danger. Remember you won't be any help to anyone if you are seriously injured while trying to rescue someone who is surrounded by danger. If you find a potential danger that you can easily handle yourself, such as pulling up the handbrake of a vehicle, or switching off the mains in the case of electrocution, don't be afraid to act swiftly if it will make the situation safer for everyone.

Next, if you are close enough, check if the person is breathing. You'll need this information for your call.

Call

Call for help as soon as possible. Gather information on the distressed person, check their pulse, the scene, and the location so you can accurately convey all this to the response team and other professionals without delay. Don't delay calling in local authorities immediately.

Care

After gathering information about the scene and state of the person, provide care until help arrives. Use the information in this book to keep the person stable and comfortable until further help arrives. Prepare to use your first aid techniques if needed. You *can* save a life.

Don't Just Stand There

During an emergency, it is easy to freeze and feel helpless. With a little bit of courage and keeping in mind your priorities, you can overcome that initial panic and slip into your role of first aider.

We understand that some of you may fear that should something go wrong during your care of the distressed person, you may be held accountable by others, including the law or courts. This is where the Good Samaritan Statute comes in. Every state has a form of good Samaritan law to encourage and enable you to offer first aid and other help, if appropriate, during emergency situations. These laws offer legal protection to those who are the first to respond to a medical emergency concerning an ill or injured person. These laws require you to act in good faith and with good intentions, act voluntarily, use common sense, and only offer help you've been trained to give. This legal coverage and situations in which care can be given varies through each state. Check your local statutes concerning these laws.

The Three Ps of First Aid

As with the Three Cs, we have the Three Ps of first aid that lay out your priorities during your care of the person requiring your assistance. These are tenets that all first aiders and paramedics subscribe to.

Preserve Life

As the first (or only) person at an emergency to offer first aid, your priority is to preserve life—in other words, keep the person alive. The goal is to prevent the decline of the person's condition. This may require you to perform an action such as CPR, stopping bleeding, or even the Heimlich Maneuver to preserve their life. Later, we will cover the A-B-C approach, also called the Circulation Method, which should be your go-to method for preserving life.

Prevent Deterioration

Your second priority is to prevent the person's condition from growing worse. This includes preventing any further injury. For instance, if the person is delirious with a fever, you may need to prevent them from moving and harming themselves even more. Other aspects of preventing deterioration may be applying first aid steps, stabilizing the person, or moving the person to a safer location if it is safe to do so. It could also mean staying with the patient to provide reassurance and comfort.

Promote Recovery

Once you've done all you can to preserve life and prevent deterioration of the person's condition, you will need to promote recovery. This can take many forms, including providing comfort and reassurance, providing temporary pain relief, if possible, and keeping the person lucid and conscious if there is a head injury.

Prepare in Advance

According to the CDC, between 2009 and 2010, about half of American adults aged 65 and over went into an emergency department. Most of them weren't prepared. (Are you prepared for a medical emergency? 2018). This lack of preparedness can create problems for doctors and first responders who have no idea what conditions they're dealing with or what medications and supplements the patients routinely take.

Preparedness is not just about prepping your family members with details of their medications lists and supplements; it also involves having a plan of action and getting into the frame of mind that prevents you from panicking at the onset.

It is natural to believe that accidents and emergencies happen to other families, or that there will always be someone else to give first aid to anyone in distress that you encounter. Given the fact that accidents and emergencies can occur at any time—day or night—and at any place to any person (even you) it's a good idea to be at least mentally prepared to act. Like in the children's book, *The Eighteenth Emergency*, what will you do if...? While the likelihood of you needing to fight off crocodiles or treat someone who's been bitten by a lion is low, chances are you could need to help someone fight a fever or treat them for a chemical burn. Instead of wondering what to do, take these few preventative steps where possible, and follow up by familiarizing yourself with the basic techniques that are in the next few chapters. Focus on following each step and you'll find that you will be able to deal with more than a few emergencies—any time, any place.

What to Prepare

- **Allocate the nearest emergency services** as a matter of course. Determine the fastest, safest route to the nearest emergency facility. Inform your family members and family carers of the services they are to use.

- **Create an Emergency Contacts List**. Have this list visible or easily at hand in the event of a crisis. Save the emergency numbers on your phone—as well as on your family members' phones, too—and instruct members when and how to contact each service. Include emergency numbers for: an ambulance service (check if your medical insurance has a specific one you should call), the fire department, the police department, your spouse, close family members and friends, dependable neighbors or nearby friends and family, and work numbers. Consider creating an emergency group on your internet messaging service with nearby friends, family, and neighbors.

- **Stock a medical kit.** You'll need to keep it up-to-date and well-stocked, replacing items as you use them. For a list of what your first aid kit should contain, see **The Contents of Your First Aid Kit**.

- **Where to find your doctor.** Know at which facilities your doctor has a practice and prioritize those locations if possible. Let caregivers and others know the name of your family doctor so it is easy to get medical histories.

- **Use medical tags.** Wear a medical tag if you suffer from any chronic conditions or uncommon allergies. Ensure family members have them, too. When assisting a person, look for a medical tag to help you give the correct information to professionals and avoid problems with medication and allergies.

- **Plan ahead.** Invest in a personal emergency response system if you are an older adult or live alone. Some security services may offer this service as an addition to their regular services. Some smartphone apps and messaging systems can also offer this function to alert friends and family. When planning travel, ensure you know where the nearest help can be located and where medical emergencies can be taken. If you are traveling abroad, be aware of regional health risks and, if need be, prepare beforehand. Don't forget to plan how to address medical emergencies arising from a family member's existing condition. Learn what their medical needs might be, ensure they have sufficient medication, particularly if you are traveling, and inform all members of the family of your response plan should an emergency arise.

- **Prepare a medical information list to assist first responders.** Include: your current and past medical conditions and surgeries; major illnesses of your immediate family (parents, siblings, children); any physical disabilities (include vision loss); names, addresses and phone numbers of your health care professionals; all of your current medication and health supplements; any legal documents for emergencies.

- We strongly recommend further study and that you certify yourself for the most used first aid techniques such as CPR.

Choosing the Proper Preparation for Your Next Actions

Keeping James Douglas' assertion in mind, it's best to take preventive measures against further harm. This simply means keeping the safety and wellbeing of all uppermost in mind. Here are some preparations and precautions you may want to take.

- Dress appropriately for cold weather. It's easy to lose body heat and sustain injuries in cold weather.

- If you are working with chemicals, prepare neutralizing solutions: an alkaline for acids and so forth.

- When traveling in hot weather and climates or water-scarce areas, carry sufficient water supplies for everyone. Ensure everyone is wearing sunblock with a high enough SPF for the time of year.

- Inform yourself about the potential risks of an activity you plan to engage in or a location you're visiting and carry the appropriate gear and supplies for emergencies.

- If you are going to do strenuous activity on vacation, get a medical check up to ensure you won't have any problems.

- If you're traveling abroad or to areas where you need malaria or other travel vaccines, ensure you and your family take these preventatives in good time.

- Be aware of any potential hazards in your area or region—severe weather, civil unrest, road closures, power and water maintenance with outages, etc., and plan accordingly.

- If you're planning on traveling to or in a remote location, ensure you and family members have sufficient chronic medication supplies to last a few extra days, or that you have a valid prescription you can easily refill.

- Monitor elderly family members and younger members for any possible adverse reactions when their medication changes. Do so over a week or more.

- Keep multipurpose salves, creams or ointments in your purse, bag, or car for small emergencies.

- Always ensure your cell phone and charger are at hand or have a power bank fully charged for emergencies.

- Carry a flashlight or mini flashlight in case of power outages or arriving late at night in ill-light areas to prevent falls and injuries.

- Ensure elderly members of the family have non-slip shoe soles.

- If you wear glasses or contacts, carry a spare pair with you.

- Wear sunglasses in strong light—summer and winter— to avoid eyestrain and injuries and accidents stemming from glare.

- Carry a spare blanket or warm covers in the car in case of a breakdown or being stranded in cold weather. In summer, have scarves or light jackets in the car.

- Ensure your vehicle is always roadworthy and that the battery is healthy.

- Ensure you and your family get enough rest during busy and stressful periods so your immunity and focus aren't compromised.

- If you are outdoors, ensure you know where the nearest running water can be found.

- Avoid food and drink from unsanitary places or that may be contaminated. Be wary of seafood left too long in the sun.

- Don't allow friends and family to drink alcohol outside in frigid weather or walk home in the cold after consuming alcohol as it could lead very quickly to hypothermia and even death.

- Never leave children, the elderly, and pets in cars when the sun is hot. Temperatures in vehicle interiors rise rapidly and can cause heat stroke or even death.

Get Your First Aid Kit Ready

It is best to keep two first aid kits—one for home and one for your car. You might want to carry a small emergency supply of pain relievers, band aids, and antacids with you to work. Tailor the kit to your needs and those of your family.

Always use the medications and preparations in your first aid kit with due care, ensuring you are using them correctly, especially if you don't use the items and preparations often. We recommend reading all ingredient labels even on over-the-counter medications as some medications may contain preservatives, sugars, or salts that may not be suitable for diabetics, people with hypertension, and people with allergies.

Assemble your kits or buy them online. If you are assembling your kit yourself, make sure your first aid bag or kit is sturdy and easily carried. It's best to keep your kit in a waterproof container or bag.

The Contents of Your First Aid Kit

A first aid kit usually contains the following items. Remember to replenish used items, and to stock quantities as per your family's needs, activities, and location. Make it a habit to go through your first aid kit periodically and replace expired contents, ensure the seals on sterile items are secure, and that your personal medications are of the correct strength as prescribed by your doctor.

Keep your first aid kits out of the reach of children and pets. Ensure older children who understand the purpose of the first aid kit know where to find it.

Your main kit should contain:

- adhesive tape

- aloe vera gel

- aluminum finger splint

- antacids

- anti-diarrhea medication

- antibiotic ointment

- antihistamine

- antiseptic solution and towelettes

- auto-injector of epinephrine if prescribed by your doctor

- bandage strips and assorted butterfly bandages

- calamine lotion

- cotton swabs and cotton-tipped swabs

- cough and cold medications

- disposable pairs of non-latex examination gloves

- duct tape

- elastic wrap bandages

- eye-shield or pad

- eyewash solution

- first aid manual

- hand sanitizer

- hydrocortisone cream

- hydrogen peroxide to disinfect

- instant cold packs

- large triangular bandage that can be used as a sling

- laxatives

- nitroglycerin

- non-stick sterile bandages and assorted roller gauze bandages

- oxymetazoline (Afrin)

- permanganate of potash

- personal medications that don't need refrigeration

- pain relievers such as acetaminophen (Tylenol) and ibuprofen (Advil, Motrin, IB)

- petroleum jelly or other lubricant

- plastic bags in assorted sizes

- plastic film

- pocket mask

- rubber tourniquet or 16 French catheter

- safety pins in assorted sizes

- scissors

- sterile saline solution for irrigation and flushing

- super glue

- surgical mask or other breathing barrier

- syringe, medicine cup, or spoon

- thermometer

- turkey baster or other suction device for flushing wounds

- tweezers

You may also keep aspirin in your first aid kit as it can be lifesaving for adults with chest pains. However, you should *never give aspirin to children*, nor use it for anyone who is allergic to it, is on blood-thinning medication, or if their doctor has advised them not to take aspirin and related medication.

We also recommend carrying a pocket mask (a mask with a tube that fits over the mouth of the person you are giving CPR) for your own safety and for easier delivery of rescue breaths.

Emergency Items

In addition to a first aid kit, you'll need some emergency items that should also be stored in waterproof, airtight containers. We recommend keeping your emergency kit with or close by your first aid kit. We suggest storing the following items.

- Emergency phone numbers including your family doctor and pediatrician, local emergency services, emergency roadside service providers, and the Poison Helpline which, in the USA, is 800-222-1222

- Medical consent forms for each family member

- Medical history forms for each family member

- Small, waterproof flashlight or headlamp with extra batteries or rechargeable

- Waterproof matches or cigarette lighter with fuel

- Safety pins to fasten bandages or slings

- Small notepad and waterproof writing instrument

- Emergency space blanket

- Cell phone with solar charger

- Sunscreen

- Insect repellent

- Water—one gallon a day for each person per a day

- Non-perishable food, including baby food if necessary

- Blanket

- Whistle

- Dust mask

- Wrench or pliers or multipurpose Swiss army knife style tool

- Plastic sheeting and duct tape for improvising shelter

- Soap, toothbrushes, feminine hygiene supplies, and other personal care items

- Moist towelettes, garbage bags, and plastic ties for personal sanitation

- Copy of Insurance cards

- Cash, change, and (if available travelers checks)

- Maps of the area

- Extra sets of car and house keys

- Personal GPS locator if you are traveling alone or hiking in remote regions.

Check your kit periodically to ensure batteries are working and safe to use, chargers are working, and items are up to date.

For Caregivers of an Aging Adult

If you are a caregiver or an aging adult, the Mayo Clinic recommends you know and note the following ten points concerning each senior. (Here are your survival kit essentials. 2019)

- Doctor's names

- Parent's birthdate

- List of allergies

- Advance directive

- Major medical problems

- List of medication and nutritional supplements

- A record of the patient's religious beliefs

- Medical insurance information

- Prior surgeries and major medical procedures

- Lifestyle information such as whether they are a teetotaler or smoker.

We strongly suggest the elderly be encouraged to prepare and execute a living will, a durable health care power of attorney, and an advance directive. The living will and advance directive record the person's preferences on medical treatment covering various circumstances. The durable health care power of attorney grants the holder authority to make medical decisions on the senior's behalf when they are unable to do so themselves. as well as allows the holder to access important medical records.

Tips for Unexpected Quarantining

Quarantining helps stop the rapid spread of an infectious disease. You may be asked to quarantine yourself, your family, or even your geographical region by your doctor, local government, or national government. Travelers may also be asked to self-isolate or quarantine to prevent any possibilities of locals being infected by a disease from another region, and vice-versa.

Quarantining can save you and others from severe illness and even death and can sometimes be imposed at very short notice. Quarantine periods may vary from seven days up to two weeks (14 days) or more. During regional quarantines, medical help may take longer to arrive, and some restrictions may apply.

If you find yourself in a sudden quarantine or needing to care for one who is self-isolating, we recommend the following.

Be Prepared at Home

If you have some notice before a quarantine is imposed:

- Ensure you have enough food and water for everyone, including your pets, for at least 14 days. It is always good to keep a few days' supply of non-perishable food such as UHT milk and canned food for any emergency, as well as ingredients to bake bread and other meal components.

- Ensure you have enough prescribed medication for all family members for two weeks.

- Ensure your first aid kits are well stocked with non-expired items, or ingredients to prepare some first aid preparations yourself.

- Have internet access, a phone, a radio, or a TV to stay updated on official news and instructions regarding a regional quarantine.

- If you are self-isolating or caring for someone in isolation, arrange to call the doctor or medical center regularly.

- Educate yourself on the signs and symptoms of the disease, as well as where and how to get help should you or anyone in your home contract the disease.

- Stock sanitizers, including extra hand sanitizers and hygiene products for everyone present.

- Stock sufficient consumables such as toilet paper, paper handkerchiefs/tissues, antibacterial wipes (or wet wipes). You may also want to include latex gloves and masks for everyone in case of having to leave your home for any reason.

- Ensure you have paracetamol to treat fevers in your first aid kits.

- Arrange with friends and family to have a buddy system in place in case your household goes into quarantine or if you live alone.

- Stock up on some wellness and activity items you and family members can do at home to keep everyone from getting cabin fever.

CHAPTER 2:

GOOD-TO-LEARN TECHNIQUES

One way to eliminate panic during a medical emergency is to learn the techniques that are used in many responses to a variety of eventualities, such as the A-B-C technique, which is used most often and in multiple circumstances. Other techniques also build up the response to effective first aid. We recommend mastering the following most employed techniques as you'll use them most often.

Before doing a diagnostic technique, keep your own safety and health in mind. You will also need to avoid cross-contamination.

If you're feeling faint or need a moment, ask for help, or take a few deep breaths and refocus on your task. Remember you're the best help the distressed person has at that moment.

While care has been taken to set out signs, symptoms, and steps to follow, your discretion and knowledge about the person in distress and other factors should also be taken into account when determining what help, if any, is required from you.

Always be aware of the dignity of the person in distress and do your best to preserve it along with their life.

Avoid Cross-Contamination and Ensure your Safety

1. Wash your hands thoroughly or use hand sanitizer or rubbing alcohol to cleanse your hands before aiding a person.

2. Don't cough, sneeze, or breathe on a wound.

3. Ensure all cuts and scrapes on your hands are covered with a waterproof dressing.

4. Wear non-latex surgical gloves and a surgical mask if they are available. If not, use plastic bags, or if the person is capable, ask them to dress their own wounds.

5. If you are giving CPR, wear a mask to avoid possible infection or contamination.

6. Don't touch a wound with your bare hands. Don't touch any part of a dressing or swab that will be directly applied to a wound.

7. Dispose of all waste carefully to reduce the risk of contamination to others. Take particular care with needles and other sharp objects. Keep them in a plastic container or similar sealed container and dispose of them with medical waste or as safely as possible.

How To Remove Objects From a Person's Pockets

Sometimes, you may need to remove a person's phone or other bulky objects from their pockets, or to search for information. To avoid complications and to reassure the person, follow these steps.

1. Ask the person for permission first.

2. If there are other people around, ask for a reliable witness.

3. Once you remove an item or the person's glasses, place it beside them where they can easily see it or find it when they recover.

4. If the person becomes unconscious, ensure all their belongings travel with them to the hospital or medical facilities or that their bundle is handed to the police.

What Information to Give When Calling Emergency Services

- Your name

- That you are responding as a first aider

- Your telephone number

- Your location

- Type of emergency

- Any details about the person in distress

- Any dangers in the area, for example, fire, smoke, live electric cables.

Keep calm and keep your answers brief and to the point. Deliver as much information as you can in the shortest possible time. Listen carefully to the dispatcher and answer clearly as best you can. It's okay if you can't answer the question, but don't waste time waffling your answers.

Taking Notes for Medical Response

As a first responder, if possible, take notes at the scene. This information will help in the fast diagnosis and treatment of the person when medical professionals arrive or when they get to a hospital.

Take note of:

- The injury or injuries found.

- How the injury occurred.

- Information the person supplies about themselves.

- Timing of events (how long between changes in conscious, changes in the person's behavior)

- The person's pulse and other vitals

- Any treatment you are giving.

- Medication used, and medication found on the person. Any medications given and time taken.

- The person's next of kin

- Your phone number.

Diagnostic Techniques

A-B-C

Once you have determined that there is no imminent environmental danger to you and the person you're assisting, and have checked whether they are responsive—responding to your voice or touch (EFWA Basic First Aid Training, 2021)—it's time to apply the A-B-C to preserve life.

A-Airway

- Is the person's airway clear? Is the person breathing?

- If the person is conscious, responding to you, and their airway is clear, assess how best you can assist them with their emergency.

- If the person is unconscious or not responding, check their airway for obstructions by opening their mouth and looking inside. If there are no obstructions, tilt their chin gently back by lifting their chin and check for breathing. If there is an **obstruction**, place the person in the **Recovery Position**, open their mouth and clear the contents, then tilt the head back and check for breathing.

B-Breathing

- Check for breathing by looking for up and down movements of the chest.

- Listen by putting your ear near their mouth or nose.

- Feel for breathing by placing your hand on the lower part of the chest.

- If the person is unconscious and breathing, carefully roll them onto their side while ensuring you keep their head, neck, and spine in alignment.

C-Circulation

- Is the person in distress bleeding profusely? If so, the bleeding must be staunched as soon as possible to prevent the person going into shock. Shock can be life-threatening, so preventing shock is a priority in preserving life.

Assess Priorities

Before applying any techniques and after checking that it's safe to offer first aid, we need to assess the priorities as the person may have more than one injury and the possibility of shock exists in most medical emergencies.

First

Identify the injuries and/or medical condition of the person. Keep in mind there might be internal injuries, particularly in the case of motor or mechanical accidents.

Second

Treat injuries in order of severity and threat to life. For instance, if a person is not breathing but is bleeding, you'll need to get them breathing first.

Third

Decide what type of care the person in distress needs. Arrange for this care by calling for help or providing comfort and reassurance until professional help arrives.

Check the Person's Response (Conscious/Unconscious)

- Determine if the person is conscious or unconscious by observing them as you approach. Next, introduce yourself even if they appear to be unconscious and unresponsive. Ask them questions or give them a command. Questions to ask might be: "What happened?" or "Are you all right?" Commands could be something like "Open your eyes!" or "Move your hand if you can hear me."

- If there is no response from the distressed person, gently shake their shoulders. If there's still no response, consider them unconscious. If the person responds by making eye contact or some other gesture, they are conscious.

Note: If you have to treat more than one person, the unresponsive or unconscious are to be attended to first. If you suspect or know that the person is a drug addict, take extra care as they may have needles on them.

Conduct the A-B-C

Run through the A-B-C diagnostic technique, clearing their airway if necessary, and shifting them into the recovery position.

Run a Secondary Survey

- Find out as much history as you can. Determine what happened and relevant medical history. You can also ask a witness if the distressed person is unconscious or cannot give a clear account. Look for medical tags and other emergency information the person might be carrying.

- Determine the symptoms—any injuries or abnormalities the person describes, or a witness provides.

- Determine the signs—injuries and abnormalities that you can see.

- Use the AMPLE method to question the person or a witness:

- A - Do you have any allergies?

- M - Do you have any medication?

- P - Do you have pre-existing conditions (hypertension, diabetes, asthma, etc.)

- L - When did you last eat, and what did you eat?

- E - Events timeline - What happened?

Keep in Mind

- Remain calm. There's no need to panic. You're doing the best you can.

- Be aware of the risks to yourself as well as to others.

- Build and maintain trust with the person you're helping.

- Remember your own needs. Ask for help even from the person you're helping, for example to clamp their hand on their wound as you prepare a sterile gauze.

Opening the Airway

- If you see a blockage at the back or high in the throat, use your finger to sweep out the obstruction. If you don't see an object, don't do a finger sweep. Be careful not to push the obstruction deeper into the airway, a hazard with younger children.

- Often, the loss of muscle control causes an airway obstruction when the tongue falls back, blocking the airway. You will want to check if the person's breathing is becoming difficult and noisy, or stopping. Lift the chin and tilt the head back as in the A-B-C to move the tongue away from the airway and allow rescue breaths to be effective.

Mouth-To-Mouth Respiration or Mouth-To-Nose Respiration for an Adult

1. Ensure the distressed person is lying flat on their back. Clear any blockage from the mouth. Kneel beside the person's head.

2. Tilt the head back.

3. Pinch the nose with one hand. With your other hand, pull their mouth open. Do not press on the neck. For mouth-to-nose respiration, close the person's mouth with your thumb.

4. Breathe in deeply. With your mouth covering the patient's mouth completely, breathe out steadily so all your breath is transferred to the patient's mouth. If you need to fill their lungs, breathe out strong breaths. Look for the patient's chest rising. For mouth-to-nose respiration, put your mouth around the person's nose.

5. Lift your mouth away, allowing the patient to breathe out and for you to take another breath of air.

6. Turn your head to look for the chest falling, feel the air they breathed out on your cheek, and to listen to the sound of the patient breathing out. For mouth-to-nose respiration, you may need to open the patient's mouth to let air out.

7. Take another breath of air. When the chest has fallen, blow into the patient's mouth or nose as you did before. Watch for the person's exhaled breath. Check that their heart is beating.

Putting Someone in the Recovery Position

1. Kneel beside the distressed person. Remove glasses and large items such as cell phones from their pockets. Don't remove smaller items from their pockets.

2. Ensure both of their legs lie straight. Lift the distressed person's arm with care and set it ninety-degrees, or as close as possible, to the body. Take care with the elbow when bending it and set the arm down with the palm facing up.

3. Move their other arm across their chest. Hold the back of their hand against their cheek closest to you. With your other hand, grasp their leg across from you just above the knee and pull it up, ensuring their foot stays flat on the ground.

4. While holding their hand against their cheek, pull on the bent leg just above the knee and roll them toward you and onto their side.

5. Adjust the upper leg (the one you pulled on), so that the hip and knee lie at ninety-degrees to each other.

6. Tilt their head back and lift their chin to prevent obstructions to their airway. If necessary, adjust their hand under their cheek to ensure the airway remains open.

7. If the person has to stay in the recovery position for more than thirty minutes, roll them onto their back, and set them in the recovery position on the other side, unless they have injuries on that side.

Cleansing and Sterilization

You'll be using two methods of cleansing and sterilizing the skin during first aid applications.

Skin Cleansing

Cleanse the skin with a swab saturated in 70 percent alcohol or organic iodine that may be labelled povidone-iodine or similar. Swipe the swab across the skin for a few seconds.

Skin Sterilization

Should you need to cut or puncture the skin, you will have to sterilize the skin so that bacteria on the skin is eliminated, except for those deep in the sweat glands and hair follicles.

However, should the person's life be threatened by a delay in treatment, skin sterilization can be skipped.

There are two methods you could use:

- Use as much 70 percent alcohol as needed to scrub the skin thoroughly for 2 minutes.

- If you have a first aid kit handy, you can apply 2% iodine tincture to a sterile gauze pad and cover the skin till the iodine dries. Use a 4x4 in2 (10x10 cm2) pad. Once you remove the pad, replace it with another gauze swab soaked in 70% alcohol to prevent the iodine from burning the skin.

When sterilizing, be sure to:

- Sterilize a much larger area of skin than at just the site of the treatment.

- When applying the disinfectant, begin where you'll be breaking the skin and work around the area in larger and larger concentric circles.

- Wear sterile gloves when disinfecting the skin.

Reducing the Risk of Infection During First Aid

- Wash or sanitize your hands using antibacterial products where possible before working on a wound.

- Wear disposable medical gloves from the first aid kit.

- Avoid breathing, coughing, and sneezing over a wound.

- Cleaning the wound depends on the type, severity of the wound, and severity of bleeding. If unsure, clean only around the wound.

- Use a sterile dressing to cover the wound. Avoid touching the surface of the dressing that is applied to the wound.

Using Bandages During First Aid

Points to remember when bandaging a distressed person include the following:

- Ensure the distressed person is seated or lying down. Move until you are in front of them, on their injured side.

- Ensure the injured body part is supported and in position before you begin bandaging.

- If the person can assist, let them hold the dressing in place as you wind the 'tail' of the bandage once fully around the limb to anchor it in place. If you have no assistance, wrap the 'tail' of the bandage directly around the padding on the wound.

- When winding the bandage around the injury, ensure every turn of the bandage overlaps the one before. An alternative method is to bandage in a "figure eight."

- To prevent circulation problems to hands and feet, ensure that the bandage is not too tight. To check that the bandage is not impeding circulation, press on a fingernail or toenail of the injured limb. If the nail quickly turns pink again, circulation is fine, and no adjustments are necessary. If the nail takes a minute or two to turn pink, or stays white, adjust the bandage as circulation is a problem. Keep doing the fingernail or toenail check as you remain with the person and adjust the bandage as needed.

CPR or Cardiopulmonary Resuscitation

Cardiopulmonary Resuscitation or CPR is a technique used to stimulate the heart and lungs.

When to Use CPR

Use CPR when the person's heart has stopped, or they are no longer breathing. CPR can also be used to help a person with distressed breathing—when they are gasping for breath.

What is CPR

CPR involves us pushing down on a person's chest and assisting with breathing by blowing air into their mouths. We do this so that blood flows to the distressed person's brain and mechanically induces blood flow to other areas of the body, thus helping to prevent brain damage and death.

Step-By-Step CPR

1. Check to see if the person is conscious.

If the person has no back or neck injury, gently shake or tap the person. Shaking someone with a spinal or head injury causes further injury. Shout "Are you okay?" If the person is not responding, move on to Step 2.

2. Start chest compressions.

For an adult or an older child who has reached puberty -

- Kneel next to the person.

- Using your fingers, locate the end of the breastbone where the ribs meet.

- Place two fingers at the tip of the breastbone.

- Place the heel of your other hand just above your fingers (pointing to the person's face)

- To compress the chest, use both hands. Remove your two fingers from the end of the breastbone and place them on top of the other hand. Then, lace your fingers and lift them so only the palms of your hands are in contact with the breastbone.

3. Position your arm and body for doing chest compressions by centering your shoulders directly above your hands on the person's chest. Straighten your arms and lock your elbows.

4. In a steady rhythm, press down using your body weight. The force of each compression should go directly onto the breastbone, depressing it at least 2 in. (5 cm). Allow the chest to re-expand after each compression.

5. If you are not trained in CPR, give at least 100 chest compressions a minute. Push hard at about one to two times a second.

6. If you are trained in CPR, start Rescue Breaths. If you are not trained in CPR, don't worry about doing Rescue Breaths, as chest compressions by themselves are effective on adults and older children. Children and babies benefit the most from rescue breathing.

7. Continue with 100 compressions a minute. Remember to allow time for the chest to expand, until the person is breathing normally.

8. If you are trained in CPR, give 30 compressions and two rescue breaths. Continue this cycle until help arrives or the person begins breathing normally.

9. When giving rescue breaths, check that the person's airway is not narrowed or blocked by an

obstruction, including the tongue, during muscle relaxation. Remember to lift the chin and tilt the head back to allow rescue breaths to travel down the airway. Exhaled air contains only about five percent less oxygen than the air we breathe in. (Piazza, et al. 2014) This is enough oxygen to supply another person with oxygen, and forcing exhaled air into their lungs could possibly save their life. Rescue breathing also forces air into the person's air passages, the air sacs in their lungs, and so into the bloodstream and into red blood cells. By removing your mouth, the person's chest can fall, exhaling air with waste products.

10. Pocket masks can be used during CPR and may be available from a first aid kit or first aid station. However, CPR should never be delayed, even to find a pocket mask.

Rescue Breaths

1. Place one hand on the person's forehead.

2. With your thumb and forefinger, pinch the person's nose closed.

3. Place the fingers of your free hand against the bone of the person's jaw and, if they have no neck injuries, tilt their chin up to ensure the airway is open.

4. Take a normal breath, seal your mouth over the person's mouth. If you are assisting with a baby,

place your mouth over the baby's mouth and nose. Blow into the person's mouth for one second, then watch to see if their chest rises.

5. If their chest does not rise, tilt their chin back and give another rescue breath.

6. Between rescue breaths, remove your mouth from the person's face and breathe normally. Allow their chest to rise and fall and feel their exhale.

Special instructions for younger children

If a young child isn't breathing:

1. Kneel by their chest or head.

2. **Using only one hand**, apply compressions to the center of the chest, not directly onto their abdomen, end of their breastbone or ribs.

3. Give 30 compressions every minute, allowing for the expansion of the chest after every compression. Don't remove your hand during the expansion of the chest.

4. When checking their airway in the CPR position, don't sweep your finger in their mouth to clear it.

5. Call for help.

6. If you are trained in giving Rescue breaths, give two breaths after every 30 compressions.

7. Continue until help arrives.

Special instructions for infant

Always stand or kneel side-on to the infant when treating them. If the infant isn't breathing:

1. Never shake the baby to check the response. Call them and flick a finger gently at the sole of their feet.

2. Check that their airway is clear:

- Roll a towel and place it under their shoulders.

- Place a finger against their forehead and push it gently back.

- With one finger on the bony part of their chin, gently tilt their chin up. Avoid touching the soft tissue under their chin as this may cut off their airway.

3. CPR for infants:

- Check their airway is clear.

- Use two straightened fingers to deliver compressions to the center of their chest.

- Ensure you depress gently to about ⅓ of their chest capacity.

- Allow their chest to expand after every compression without removing your fingers.

- Give 30 compressions at a rate of 100 compressions a minute.

- Check their airway. Remove any visible objects. Don't sweep your finger in their mouth to clear out objects as it may deliver the object into their throats.

   4. Hold the infant in the recovery position: cradle the baby with their head to the side lower than their torso.

Special instructions for Pregnant Women

When setting a pregnant woman on the ground to do the A-B-C, CPR or in the recovery position, elevate her right hip with tightly packed rolled-up towels or clothing if there is no one to help you.

When placing her in the recovery position, roll her onto her left side.

The Heimlich Maneuver

You may have heard of this technique before. It is also called Abdominal Thrusts.

When to Use the Heimlich Maneuver

Use the Heimlich Maneuver when a person is choking.

How to Perform the Heimlich Maneuver

Performing the Heimlich Maneuver on a person in distress -

1. Stand behind the person, or kneel behind them if they are a child. Keep one of your feet slightly ahead of the other to balance yourself. Wrap your arms around their waist and tip the person slightly forward.

2. With one hand, make a fist and place it just above their navel.

3. With your other hand, grasp your fist. Press hard into their abdomen in a fast, upward motion as if you're trying to lift them off the ground.

4. Repeat the maneuver six to ten times until their airway is cleared of the blockage.

Taking a Pulse (Heart Rate)

The rate at which your heart beats is called a pulse. A pulse can be felt in certain locations of the body where larger blood vessels are close to the skin's surface—areas such as your wrist and neck.

The standard pulse for an adult not exerting themselves is usually between 60 to 100 beats per minute. Your pulse may change in times of illness, so it is important to know your usual pulse when you are generally fit and healthy. To find your resting pulse or usual pulse, take your pulse only after you've been sitting or resting quietly for about five minutes. However, in the case of an emergency, a pulse should be taken immediately.

How to Take Your Pulse

Check your pulse on the inside of your wrist.

- Place two fingers on the artery below your thumb to feel your pulse. Always use your fingers and never your thumb as your thumb has its own pulse that will make counting beats difficult.

- Use a light, gentle touch so you can detect even a light pulse.

- Count the beats for 30 seconds, then multiply by two to get the beats per minute—your pulse rate.

- You can also record if your pulse is strong or weak, and regular or irregular.

How to Take Someone's Pulse

- For babies, take their brachial pulse by placing two fingers on the inner side of their upper arm. For older children, you can take their radial pulse at the wrist or their carotid pulse at the hollow of their neck and clavicle. Their pulse rate should be higher than a healthy adult but still within the 60-100 beats per minute rate.

- For an adult, you can place two fingers on their wrist or their carotid artery on their neck to find their pulse. If the person is fit, their pulse rate may be slower.

Splinting

A splint is used to prevent further injury to an arm, leg, fingers or toes that may be severely sprained, fractured, or broken by immobilizing it until professional help arrives. A splint may also be useful in the event of a snakebite while awaiting help.

How to Splint a Limb

Use one of two methods -

1. Tie the injured arm or leg to a stiff, sturdy object. your aim is to prevent the limb bending, so any stiff object of a suitable length will do, such as a stick, a cane, or even rolled up magazines and newspapers. Use a belt, a rope, a bandage, or another suitable item to tie the splint securely to

the limb. Ensure that the splint is not too tight and does not impede circulation and that it prevents any bending of the limb.

2. Secure the injured finger, toe, or limb to another part of the body. For example, you may tape an injured finger to the finger adjacent to it or fasten an injured arm so it is held against the chest. Ensure the splint is not too tight and is not causing further injury or discomfort to the person.

In the event of a fracture or snakebite, splinting is only an emergency measure. Professional health care must be sought immediately.

Rules to Observe While Splinting

- Splint a limb from the joint above an injury to the joint below the injury. For example, splint a broken shin from above the knee to the ankle.

- If you have to transport the person a long or difficult distance, additional support to splints may be required.

- Never secure the splint directly over the injury, i.e. never tie ropes, belts or other fasteners directly over a fracture or snakebite.

- Always ensure that the splint, while securely fastened, never affects circulation. Do the fingernail test to check if circulation remains healthy.

- In some cases, swelling may occur over the injury. Adjust the splint by loosening it to ensure that circulation is not cut off.

- Always use padding when splinting knees and ankles if they are tied together.

Slings

A sling is often used to immobilize an arm in the case of a suspected fracture (including rib fracture), dislocation, or other injuries. A sling's function is to hold the injured arm, bent at the elbow, comfortably across the person's torso. Usually, the hand of the bent arm, points upwards towards the opposite shoulder as the sling supports the weight of the forearm.

If no slings or triangular bandages are available, then a sling can be easily improvised using clothing for a short-term measure until medical help and a sturdier sling can be used.

Note: Once in a sling, it is important to regularly check circulation by noting the color of the person's fingernails (they should be healthy pink) and ensuring the person's arm doesn't begin to tingle or feel numb.

Improvising Slings

- **Use a jacket or button-up coat.** Undo the button of a coat, waistcoat, or jacket around the person's chest. Slip in their arm, resting their wrist on the button beneath. Alternatively, use the corner of the jacket. Undo the jacket fastening. Fold the bottom end up and over the injured arm forming a cradle for the arm. Pin the edge of the jacket to the person's shoulder with safety pins. Tuck in any edges.

- **If the person is using a long-sleeved shirt,** position their injured arm across their chest with elbow bent, pin the cuff of the shirt to their breast. Alternatively, pin their cuff to their shoulder if an elevated sling is needed.

- **Use a belt, long, thin scarf, a tie, etc.** to create a looped sling. Create a loop with the belt or scarf (tie or fasten the ends together) and hang it around the person's neck. Twist the lower end of the loop to create a lower loop (the item will now be in a figure eight) and slip the person's hand through the lower-loop. Avoid this method if you suspect a wrist injury.

- **Use a meter square of strong material or a large square scarf.** Fold the material into a triangle (bring diagonally opposite ends together), and knot at the shoulder to form a cradle for the arm. Ensure the knot is safe and secure—square knots are best—and that the person's arm is comfortable. Tuck in the material ends by the elbow.

Treating Convulsions and Fits

1. If the person is convulsing, lie them on their back in a safe place free of sharp and hard objects.

2. Turn the person onto their side so that their tongue moves to the front of the mouth and froth can freely flow out of their mouth.

3. Place a folded cloth under the person's head or hold their head so that they don't injure themselves from banging their head.

4. Allow the person to move their arms and legs, and to shake.

5. Loosen tight clothing.

Don't try to open the person's mouth or place anything in it.

Handing Over to Paramedics

When paramedics or other professional medical personnel arrive:

- continue assisting the person in distress until the paramedics ask you to step aside

- tell the medical personnel all that you can, including details of the injury, your treatment, and details about medication

- assist the paramedics further until they ask you to step aside

- hand your notes to the paramedics

- ensure all the person's belongings are in their care or that of the paramedic crew.

CHAPTER 3:

MILD EMERGENCIES

Not all emergencies may be a risk to life, yet they can be overwhelming to deal with if you aren't sure how to treat them. Most common emergencies not requiring urgent medical attention occur at home, while traveling, during leisure activities—almost anywhere and at any time. Let's look at how to treat some common emergencies without calling for medical assistance from the outset.

Bites and Stings

Almost everyone will experience bites and stings, particularly when outdoors and during spring and summer. Most bites and stings can be quickly and efficiently treated. However, stings in the mouth, throat or multiple stings must be medically treated as they obstruct the airways and are more likely to lead to anaphylaxis.

What Not to Do

The following will cause infection and intensify the effects of the venom. You may also harm yourself in the process.

1. Don't cut into the wound or cut it out.

2. Don't attempt to suck venom out of a wound.

3. Don't use a tourniquet or tight bandage.

4. Don't treat the wound with chemicals or medicines (for example, potassium permanganate crystals) or inject into the wound.

5. Don't put ice packs on the wound.

6. Don't use proprietary snake bite kits.

Applying traditional and herbal remedies on severe stings and bites may not be of much help and can even be life-threatening. It may be better to find professional medical assistance or hospitalization as soon as possible.

General Rules to Treat Bites and Stings

Your priority: Keep the person calm and still, prevent rapid swelling, arrange transport and care to a medical facility.

1. Reassure and comfort the distressed person. Most people will panic when stung or bitten. In a calm voice, explain that most bites and stings from insects, spiders, snakes, and sea creatures are harmless, and even dangerous creatures seldom carry poison that harms humans.

2. While keeping the person calm, keep them still with the injured body part below the level of the heart. Movement, particularly of an injured limb, and fear and excitement spread the venom quickly and worsens the person's condition. Consider using a splint to immobilize a bitten arm or leg.

3. Remove the person's rings, watch, bracelets, anklets, and shoes, and loosen restrictive clothing if there is swelling.

4. The patient should lie on one side in the recovery position to ensure their airway is clear and in case of fainting or vomiting.

5. Do not feed the person anything by mouth—food, alcohol, medicines, or drinks—unless there is a delay in getting medical care or the risk of dehydration. Then, only allow the person water.

6. If the person has been stung in the mouth or throat, give them an ice cube to suck or let them sip ice water to reduce swelling and keep their airway open until help arrives.

7. Try to identify the animal that caused the wound, but don't attempt to capture or hold the creature if this may put you and others at risk. If the animal is dead, take it to the hospital with the person, but handle it with great care as even dead animals may still inject venom.

8. Arrange to transport the person to a hospital, a clinic, or another professional medical center as soon as possible. Ensure that the person remains as still as possible. Don't allow the person to walk. If no ambulance or other vehicle is available, carry them on a stretcher or a makeshift one. If a bicycle is available, carry them across the handlebar of the bike.

9. Antivenom, if available, should only be administered if there is evidence of severe poisoning, and in a location where resuscitation can be given, such as a medical center or hospital as the person may experience an allergic reaction. Antivenom must not be used if there are no signs of poisoning.

Dog and Cat Bites

Cat and dog bites usually leave small puncture wounds. However, if there's a tearing of flesh, medical care must be sought.

Treating Dog and Cat Bites

Your priority: Cleanse the wound, prevent inflammation and infection, and seek medical help if you suspect the animal is ill.

1. Wash the wound with water to remove the bacteria-rich saliva of the animal.

2. Keep the bitten area lower than the heart, if possible.

3. Bathe the wound in a mild solution of permanganate of potash.

4. Apply a clean dressing.

If you suspect the animal is rabid, seek medical help immediately.

Spider Bites

Spider bites seldom cause major injury. However, venomous spiders such as black widow spider and the brown recluse spider can be quite dangerous.

Seek immediate medical help when:

- The bite is from a black widow or brown recluse spider.

- You're not sure if the spider might be poisonous.

- The person has a growing ulcer at the site of the bite or severe abdominal cramping.

- The person isn't breathing.

Treating Spider Bites

Your priority: Cleanse the wound. Prevent inflammation and infection.

1. Cleanse the wound using mild soap and water. Apply an antibiotic ointment.

2. If the bite is on an arm or leg, elevate the limb. Apply a cool compress to reduce pain and swelling. Dampen a cloth with cold water or fill the cloth with ice.

3. Over-the-counter pain medication can be used for further pain management, and, if the wound is itchy, an antihistamine (Benadryl, Chlor-Trimeton, etc.) may help.

4. A tetanus shot may be needed if the person bitten has not had one in five years.

Snake Bites

Despite common perception, only about 15% of snakes worldwide are a danger to humans.

Treating Snake Bites

Your priority: Seek medical help, move the person away from the snake, cleanse the bite.

While waiting for medical help:

1. Move out of the snake's striking distance.

2. Remain calm and still to prevent fast dispersion of the venom into the bloodstream.

3. Discard jewelry and tight clothing before swelling begins.

4. Position the person, if possible, so that the bite is below or at the level of the heart.

5. Cleanse the bite with soap and water.

6. Cover the bite with a clean, dry dressing.

What Not to Do:

- Don't apply ice or use a tourniquet.

- Don't attempt to remove the venom by cutting the wound or sucking on the bite.

- Don't allow the person bitten any caffeine or alcohol as these quicken the body's absorption of venoms.

- Don't attempt to capture the snake. Try to remember its color and shape, and other distinguishing features you can describe that will help in identification for treatment. If you have your smartphone handy and it is safe to do so, take a photo of the snake for easier identification.

Human Bites

Human bites can be even more dangerous than most animal bites as the human mouth contains vast amounts of bacteria and viruses. Human bites that break the skin can therefore become infected. When someone's knuckles are cut by another person's teeth (as may happen in a fight) this, too, is considered a human bite. When you do the same to yourself during a fall or accident, it is also considered a human bite.

Treating Human Bites

Your priority: Stop the bleeding. Seek medical care.

1. Stop bleeding by applying pressure with a clean, dry cloth.

2. Wash the wound thoroughly with soap and water.

3. Cover the wound with non-stick, clean bandage.

4. Seek medical care.

5. If the person bitten hasn't had a tetanus shot in five years, a booster shot may be needed within 48 hours of the bite.

Stings

Insect stings seldom cause major injury, but they can cause severe pain, particularly if the sting is on the lips or mouth.

Treating Stings

Your priority: Remove the sting. Prevent inflammation and infection.

1. If a sting is from a bee, hornet, wasp, or similar insect, remove the thorny sting with a pair of tweezers. If no tweezers are available, apply pressure around the sting to force it up and out, or use a plastic card such as a credit card to scrape it off by scraping from the thorny side.

2. Wash the wound thoroughly with soap and water. If available, apply an ointment or lotion to relieve itching.

3. Caution the person not to scratch the sting as this can cause infection.

Choking

A person chokes when an object obstructs their windpipe and interferes with their breathing, usually causing them a severe shortage of breath.

Signs and Symptoms

- Most people will clutch their throat when choking

- An inability to talk

- Labored or noisy breathing

- Squeaky sounds when trying to breathe

- Coughing that's weak or forceful

- Skin, lips, or nails turning dusky or blue

- Flushed skin that soon turns pale or bluish

- Loss of consciousness

Treating Someone Who Is Choking

Your priority: Dislodging the blockage as quickly as possible, assisting with breathing if necessary.

1. If the person can cough strongly, encourage them to cough the obstruction out.

2. Dislodge the object in their throat by leaning their head and shoulders forward and thump their back hard between the shoulder blades. If a child is choking, hold them upside down and thump their backs between the shoulder blades.

3. If the person cannot cry, laugh hard, or talk, the American Red Cross recommends the Five-and-Five approach to assist the distressed person:

a) Thump the person's back 5 times.

b) Stand to the side and just behind a choking adult. If it is a child choking, kneel behind them. Place one hand across their chest for support. Bend the person's waist

70

as you thump them between the shoulder blades with the heel of your hand.

c) Perform five Abdominal Thrusts, also known as the Heimlich Maneuver.

d) Alternate between five thrusts and five abdominal thrusts until the object is dislodged.

4. If you are alone and choking, you can perform abdominal thrusts on yourself by:

a) Placing your fist just above your navel.

b) Grasping your fist with your other hand and bending over a hard surface such as a desk, chair, or countertop.

c) Shoving your fist inward and upward.

5. To clear the airway of a pregnant or obese person:

a) During the Heimlich Maneuver, position your hands a little higher, just under the breastbone and the conjunction of the lowest ribs.

b) Perform the Heimlich Maneuver with a quick thrust.

c) Repeat until the object is dislodged from the throat.

6. If the person becomes unconscious. Perform the following steps.

a) Lower the person to the floor on their back with their arms to the side.

b) Clear the airway as in the A-B-C.

c) Begin CPR if the person remains unresponsive and the object remains lodged in their airway. The chest compressions may dislodge the obstruction.

d) Check the mouth often to ensure their airway remains clear and for the dislodged object.

7. To clear the airway of an infant who is not yet a year old:

a) Sit down. Hold the infant across your forearm. Rest your forearm on your thigh. Support the baby's head and neck with your hand and place their head lower than their trunk.

b) Using the heel of your hand, gently thump their back between the shoulder blades five times. Keep your fingers pointed up, so you don't hit the infant's head. Gravity and your blows combined should dislodge the object.

c) If the infant is still not breathing, turn the infant face-up on your forearm, supported by your thigh with their head lower than their trunk. Use two fingers placed on the center of their breastbone, give five quick compressions. Press down about 1.5 inches and allow the chest to rise in between compressions.

d) If breathing doesn't resume, repeat the back blows and chest compressions. Call for medical help.

e) Do <u>Infant CPR</u> if the object dislodges but the infant doesn't begin breathing.

8.
If the child is older than a year old and conscious, administer the <u>Heimlich Maneuver</u>, taking care not to use too much force as this can injure the child's ribs and internal organs.

Eye Trauma

When foreign bodies enter the eye, they can cause discomfort in the eyeball and eyelid. If the foreign body becomes embedded in the eyeball, it can cause severe problems.

Treating Eye Trauma

Your priority: Prevent further injury to the eye, remove irritants safely, promote recovery of the eye.

1. Prevent the person from rubbing their eye. Position them so that they are facing your light and you can stand in front of them.

2. Pull down their lower eyelid. With the corner of a clean cloth or handkerchief (white, twirled up, and moistened, if possible) remove the foreign object.

3. If the object is embedded, don't attempt to remove the object. Have the person close their eye and apply a soft pad of cotton wool secured with a bandage.

4. If the foreign body is not found and you suspect that it lies under the upper eyelid, encourage the person to blink underwater. Alternatively, lift the upper eyelid forward, push the lower lid below it and release both lids simultaneously. The lower lid lashes may brush out the object from the upper eyelid.

5. If a liquid irritant is in the eye, get the person to blink underwater or flush the eyes out with copious amounts of water. Apply a soft cotton pad over the eye kept in position by a pair of shades or a lightly fixed bandage.

Nosebleed

A common emergency in anyone of any age, nosebleeds are usually not a true medical problem, but can sometimes indicate a severe problem.

Treating Nosebleeds

Your priority: Stop the nosebleed by pinching the nostrils shut.

1. Sit the person down and lean their head forward to reduce blood pressure in the nose and to discourage further bleeding. This position prevents them from swallowing blood which can cause stomach irritation.

2. Get the person to gently blow their nose to clear blood clots in their nose. Spray both sides of the nose with a nasal decongestant with oxymetazoline (Afrin).

3. Pinch their nostrils shut using your thumb and forefinger. Instruct them to breathe through their mouth. Keep their nose pinched shut for about 10 to 15 minutes. This often stops the bleeding as it puts pressure on the point of the nose that is bleeding.

4. If the nosebleed persists after 10 to 15 minutes, continue pinching their nose shut for another 10 to 15 minutes. Avoid looking into the nose. If the bleeding still hasn't stopped, get emergency medical care.

5. Advise the person with the nosebleed to avoid blowing or picking their nose, and avoid bending down, for several hours. Keep their head higher than their heart. If available, apply petroleum jelly

gently into the nostrils using a cotton swab or a finger.

6. If the bleed resumes, repeat the steps above, but if the nosebleed persists, get medical care as soon as possible.

Fainting

Fainting occurs when a person's brain experiences a temporary shortage of blood resulting in a brief loss of consciousness. A faint can have little medical significance, or it can be an indicator of a serious medical condition, usually involving the heart.

Treating Fainting

Your priority: Keeping the person still and out of danger. Assist with breathing if necessary.

If you feel faint:

1. Lie down or sit down.

2. If you're sitting down, place your head between your legs for a minute or two.

3. Avoid fainting again by slowly and cautiously getting up. Keep your movements slow.

If someone else faints:

1. Set the person on their back.

2. Loosen restrictive clothing such as ties, scarfs, collars, and belts.

3. If they aren't injured and they're breathing, raise their legs above their heart level—about 12 inches or 30 centimeters.

4. Don't allow the person to get up quickly or too soon to avoid them fainting again.

5. Check the person's breathing. If they stop breathing, perform CPR.

Headaches

Most headaches are minor emergencies and don't require medical attention. However, sometimes a headache can indicate quite serious conditions. Serious or dangerous headaches are often unexplained and persistent. Get medical advice or care as soon as possible in those cases.

Headaches can be treated with pain relievers. Alternative remedies are also possible treatments. Consult **Chapter 6**.

Migraines

Migraines are quite common, particularly in women.

Signs and Symptoms of Migraines

- Causes moderate to severe pain, stemming from one or more triggers

- Pulsates or throbs

- Causes nausea, vomiting, increases sensitivity to light and sound.

- Usually affects one side of the head but can affect both sides.

- Worsens with activity such as climbing steps

- Lasts four to 72 hours without treatment

Treating Migraines

The aim of treating a migraine is to alleviate the symptoms and avoid extending the migraine attack.

If migraine triggers are known, migraine management and avoiding or alleviating triggers is crucial to reduce the severity and duration of a migraine. Treatment may take various forms or combinations of individual treatments.

Treatments may include:

- Rest in a quiet, dark room

- Applying hot or cold compresses to the back of the head or neck.

- Massage and small amounts of caffeine if the person is not a heavy coffee-drinker.

- Over-the-counter painkillers such as ibuprofen (Advil, Motrin, etc.), aspirin (if the person isn't on blood thinning medication or allergic to it), and acetaminophen (Tylenol and others).

- Preventive and prescription medication such as metoprolol (Lopressor), propranolol (Innopran, Inderal, etc., amitriptyline, divalproex (Depakote), topiramate (Qudexy XR, Trokendi XR, Topamax, erenumab-aooe (Aimovig)

Foodborne Illness

Foodborne illness often occurs when the natural bacteria in all food multiplies excessively when food is not cooked, cleaned, or stored properly. Food can also be contaminated by chemicals, toxins, viruses, and parasites.

Signs and Symptoms

- Diarrhea, often turning bloody

- Nausea

- Abdominal pain

- Vomiting

- Dehydration

- Low-grade fever at times

Excessive dehydration can result in further symptoms:

- Feeling faint of light-headed, particularly when upright

- Tiredness

- Dark-colored urine

- Less frequent urination

- Excessive thirst

Treating Foodborne Illnesses

Your priority: Ensure the person is hydrated.

1. Let the person slowly sip liquids (water or sports drinks with electrolytes). This prevents dehydration and sipping, instead of ingesting large amounts of liquids at once, and prevents vomiting and nausea.

2. Look for signs of dehydration. Monitor urination. Infrequent and dark urine instead of frequent clear urine indicates dehydration. Feeling faint

and dizzy are also signs of dehydration. If these signs appear despite hydrating as best you can, seek medical attention.

3. Anti-diarrheal medication must be avoided as they prevent or slow the cause of the diarrhea (organisms or toxins) being expelled from the body. You may want to check with a doctor if you are unsure how to proceed.

Foreign Objects in the Nose

A foreign object in the nose can be very painful.

Removing a Foreign Object from a Nose

Your priority: Avoiding further injury to the nose while gently coaxing out the object without force.

1. Don't probe for the object in the nose with a cotton swab.

2. Ask the person to not inhale the object any further, and to breathe through the mouth until their nose is clear.

3. Instruct them to blow their nose gently and calmly, without force and not in quick succession. If only one nostril is affected by the object, instruct the person to hold their clear nostril shut and commence breathing gently and calmly.

4. When the object is visible and may be easily reached and gripped by tweezers, gently remove the foreign object. Never attempt to remove an object you cannot see.

Foreign Object in the Ear

A foreign object in the ear is not only painful, but can also cause a loss of hearing and infection.

Removing a Foreign Object from an Ear

Your priority: Avoiding further injury and coaxing the object out of the ear by one of the following methods.

1. Avoid probing the ear with a cotton swab or other tool as you may push the object further into the ear canal and risk injury to the person.

2. If the object can be easily seen, easily reached and gripped with tweezers, and is pliant, gently remove it.

3. If the object cannot be seen, utilize gravity. Tip the person's head to the side with the affected ear pointing to the ground. Allow the object to fall out, if possible.

4. If the foreign object is an insect, use warm (not hot) oil to float the insect out of the ear by tilting the person's head with the affected ear facing up towards the light. Use baby oil, olive oil, or mineral

oil. Only use this method to remove insects from ears. If you suspect the person's eardrum may be perforated or you are assisting a child with ear tubes, don't use this method. Signs of a perforated eardrum include bleeding, pain, and a discharge from the ear.

5. Irrigate the ear with warm water using a bulb syringe to wash the object out of the ear. Don't use this method if the person has ear tubes in place or you suspect they may have a perforated eardrum.

Fever

When our body temperature rises above 100.4 F or 38 C, we have a fever. Fevers are often a sign of infection and most fevers we experience are not harmful. In many cases, they are helpful in fighting off an infection. Most fevers don't require medical treatment. However, some fevers over an extended period can be debilitating, or even fatal if no medical care is given. It is therefore wise to monitor fevers.

How to Check for a Fever:

- Internal temperature (ear, rectal, or temporal artery temperature) is 100.4 F (38 C) or higher.

- Oral temperature is 100 F (37.8 C) or higher.

- Armpit temperature is 99 F (37.2 C) or higher.

Treating Fevers

Your goal is to promote rest and relieve discomfort.

For adults:

1. Ensure the person stays hydrated by drinking plenty of liquids.

2. Encourage them to dress in lightweight clothing.

3. Cover them with a light blanket if they experience chills. Once the chills end, remove the blanket.

4. Take acetaminophen (Tylenol, etc.) or ibuprofen (Advil, etc). Always follow the recommended dosage.

For children:

1. Ensure the child drinks plenty of liquids.

2. Encourage them to wear lightweight clothing.

3. If the child experiences the chills, cover them with a light blanket.

4. Never give aspirin to children or teens.

5. Don't give infants pain relievers.

6. If the child is 6 months or older, give them a child's dosage of acetaminophen (Tylenol, etc.) or ibuprofen (Advil, etc.). Always read the instructions and dosage before administering the medication.

Sunburn

We've all experienced sunburn after prolonged exposure to the sun. Sunburnt skin turns red, is painful and swollen. Sometimes, blisters may appear. Headaches, fever, and nausea often accompany sunburn.

Treat Sunburn

Your priority: Cool the skin, apply a soothing gel or cream, and hydrate the person.

1. Cool the skin by bathing in cool water or applying a cool compress by wetting a clean, soft towel in cold water.

2. Apply a moisturizer, gel, or lotion preferably containing calamine or aloe vera, both of which soothe the skin.

3. Ensure the person drinks plenty of water to stay hydrated.

4. Don't break any blisters that may form. If blisters burst, cleanse the skin gently with a mild soap and water. Apply an antibiotic ointment. Cover

the area with a non-stick gauze bandage. Should a rash develop, stop using the ointment and seek medical care.

5. Pain relievers such as ibuprofen (Advil, Motrin, IB, etc.) may be taken and may ease swelling. Other pain-relieving medications for sunburn may take the form of gels.

6. Keep the person out of the sun as their skin heals.

7. Apply an over-the-counter hydrocortisone cream for severe sunburn.

Gastroenteritis

Gastroenteritis occurs when your intestines and stomach become inflamed. Symptoms can last from a day to more than a week, depending on the cause of the inflammation. Viruses and contaminated food or water are the most common causes of gastroenteritis. Side effects from a medication is another common cause of this illness.

Signs and Symptoms of Gastroenteritis:

- Nausea or vomiting

- Cramps

- Diarrhea

- Low grade fever in some cases

Treating Gastroenteritis

Your priority: Ensure the person is hydrated. Monitor their condition.

1. To avoid dehydration, ensure the person drinks lots of liquids, particularly water, sports drinks, and other electrolyte replacement drinks. Encourage them to sip the liquids for some time as ingesting large amounts of liquids all at once may cause vomiting and nausea.

2. Monitor urination to guard against dehydration. The person should frequently be urinating with light to clear urine. Dark urine passed infrequently is a major sign of dehydration. Ask the person if they feel light-headed or dizzy. These are also signs of dehydration. If these signs appear despite their hydrating well, seek medical attention.

3. Slowly introduce small amounts of bland, easy to digest food. Encourage the person to eat small portions frequently to avoid nausea. Offer foods such as soda crackers, toast, gelatin, bananas, applesauce, rice, and chicken. If the person experiences nausea once again, stop serving food and resume the liquids. Alcohol, dairy, caffeine, nicotine, fatty foods, and spicy food are to be avoided for a few days.

4. Encourage the person to rest as their bodies will be depleted and they will experience fatigue.

Sprains

Between your joints lie ligaments, elastic-like structures that connect and allow the bones to work together. When the fibers of a ligament are torn in an injury, we call it a sprain.

The most common type of sprain is an ankle sprain. Knee, wrist, and thumb sprains are also common.

Signs of a sprain include rapid swelling and pain and difficulty moving the joint.

Treating Sprains

Your priority: Keeping the person's weight off the limb and prevent swelling by icing the sprain.

1. Keep the person's weight off their limb and rest the limb for at least 48 to 72 hours. This may mean the person must use a crutch, a splint, or a brace. However, activity should not be avoided.

2. Apply ice or a cold compress to limit swelling. A slush bath, cold pack, or a compression sleeve filled with cold water can be used. Ice the injury as soon as possible for at least 15 to 20 minutes. During the next 48 to 72 hours, periodically ice the injury four to eight times a day until the swelling subsides. When using ice, be careful not

to use it for long periods as this causes tissue damage.

Sprains can take days to months to recover. Once the pain and swelling subsides, encourage the person to use the limb gently and with caution. They should experience gradual progress. However, care must be taken not to overtax the injured area and cause a repeat sprain.

Hyperventilation

Hyperventilation is rapid breathing, often quite deep breathing which results in too little carbon dioxide in the body. This may lead to dizziness, tingling of the limbs, excessive sweating, and trembling. The person's pulse rate will also be very high.

Hyperventilation usually accompanies panic attacks but can also be the result of a medical condition, and emotional upset. Most children tend to hyperventilate due to emotional upset or a medical condition.

Treating Hyperventilation

Your priority: Calming the person down. Helping them seek medical advice.

1. Speak firmly and kindly to the person.

2. Remove them from the upset or lead them to a quiet, open space.

3. Coach them to take slower breaths. If it helps, ask them to sit with their head between their knees for a minute or two.

4. Do not allow the person to breathe into a paper bag and rebreathe their expelled air as it could cause more harm if they have an infection.

CHAPTER 4:

SERIOUS EMERGENCIES

Serious emergencies require swift attention. You will now learn the necessary actions to deal rapidly with unexpected emergencies that include shock, burns, cuts, and wounds. You will also learn to attend to various outdoor emergencies such as heat stroke, hypothermia, frostbite, fractures, and even electrocution. Remember, the less you panic and follow the steps in order, the more likely the situation will remain manageable until help arrives.

NB! Take care with the medications you give a distressed person. You are not allowed to give your own prescription medications or even direct someone else to go to a pharmacy to procure your own preference of a medication to be administered. Only use medication from a first aid kit in their recommended dosage.

Shock

Shock is an indicator that a person's body is shutting down functions. This happens when your body cannot send enough blood to vital organs like the heart and brain.

Shock can be caused by sudden injury, illness, bleeding, and even emotional distress. Mild injury can also cause shock.

Symptoms of Shock

Adults and children may show the following symptoms:

- Fainting or falling unconscious

- Feeling faint, dizzy, or extremely light-headed

- Feeling very weak and losing motor-control, such as having trouble standing.

- Lack of alertness or feeling that they cannot think clearly. This may appear as confusion, fear, restlessness, or being unresponsive to questions.

Babies and younger children may show the following symptoms:

- Losing consciousness or passing out

- Extreme sleepiness or they are hard to wake up

- Unresponsive to touch or talk

- Hyperventilating

- Confusion. They may be unaware of their surroundings or unable to express where they are.

Treating Shock

Your priority: Treat any bleeding, assist with breathing if necessary, ensure the person is warm and reassured.

1. Act promptly as this could save their life.

2. Get the person to lie down. In the event of a head, neck, or chest injury, keep their legs flat. If there is no such injury, raise their legs about 12 inches or 30 centimeters.

3. If the person vomits, roll them onto their side to drain their mouth. If you suspect the person has a chest, neck or head injury, gently roll their head, neck, shoulders and body together as a unit using the log roll technique from the A-B-C.

4. Stop any bleeding.

5. Splint any broken bones.

6. Ensure the person is warm, but not hot. In a cold environment, put a blanket under them and cover them with another blanket or a sheet. In a hot environment, keep the person cool and shaded from the sun.

7. Take the person's pulse.

8. Keep the person calm until they recover, or medical help arrives.

Smoke Inhalation

If a person has inhaled smoke or fumes, they will have little oxygen in their body and may need help breathing. Besides smoke, most fires release toxic fumes from burnt plastics and other items, causing more respiratory problems and even poisoning.

If someone has passed out from fumes or smoke in an enclosed area, don't attempt to rescue them without first using appropriate breathing gear as you will most likely be overcome by the smoke or fumes yourself.

If a person is in a garage with a vehicle engine running, they will most likely have carbon monoxide poisoning. Open the garage first before attempting to help them.

Signs and Symptoms of Smoke and Fumes Inhalation:

- Coughing

- Hoarse breathing and shortness of breath

- Smarting and red, irritated eyes

- Tightness in chest and chest pains

- Headache

- Drowsiness and confusion

- Irregular or rapid pulse

- Soot in the mouth and nose

- Burns on skin or skin has a bluish tinge

- Nausea or vomiting (particularly with carbon monoxide poisoning)

Treating Smoke Inhalation

Your priority: Call emergency services, help the person to find oxygen and breathe normally.

1. Call emergency services, telling them the nature of the fire or the fumes.

2. If it's safe for you to do so, help the person into an area away from the fire or fumes where there is clean air.

3. If their clothes are on fire, have them drop and roll on the ground.

4. If the person loses consciousness and stops breathing, give CPR.

5. Coach the person to breathe normally.

6. Treat any burns.

7. Stay with the person until medical help arrives. Anyone who experiences smoke inhalation must be treated by a doctor as some effects can persist

for days, even months, and symptoms can be delayed.

Common and Chemical Burns and Scalds

Most burns, whether sustained at work or at home, tend to be minor injuries. When burnt by a hair appliance, hot stove, or hot water, home treatment is sufficient to treat the burn to avoid infection and promote healing.

Less common burns can result from dry heat such as hot metal, fire, contact with highly charged electrical current or friction from fast moving items such as rope or cloth. Burns can also result from mechanical devices such as revolving wheels, and corrosive chemicals that are strong acids or alkali.

A scald occurs when a person is injured by moist heat such as hot water, steam, hot oil, or tar.

Types of Burns

Heat or thermal burns are caused by hot objects, hot liquids, fire, or steam. Scald burns from hot liquids and steam are the most common type of burn.

Cold temperature burns are caused when exposed skin is damaged by wet, windy, or cold conditions.

Electrical burns are caused when a person is harmed by contact with electrical sources or lightning.

Chemical burns are caused by contact with household or industrial chemicals in a liquid, gas, or solid form. Natural foods, such as chili peppers, contain substances that cause skin irritation and a burning sensation.

Radiation burns are caused by the sun, sunlamps, tanning booths, X-rays, or radiation treatment for cancer.

Friction burns result from friction from hard surfaces such as roads (road rash), carpets, or gym floors. These tend to be a combination of a scrape and a heat burn, Athletes may experience friction burns from floors, courts, or tracks when they fall. Bicycle and motorcycle riders without protective clothing may experience friction burns if they fall.

Effects and Signs

Scalds and burns have the same effect. This may range from a reddening of the skin, blistering, destruction of the skin, and deeper tissue damage.

Burn Degrees

The seriousness of a burn depends on its depth (damage to skin and inner tissue) and size of the area burnt.

- First degree burns harm only the first layer of skin.

- Second degree burns fall into two categories:

1. Superficial partial-thickness burns injure the first and second layers of skin.

2. Deep partial thickness burns damage deeper layers of skin.

- Third degree burns damage all the layers of the skin as well as the tissue beneath. These burns must receive professional medical care.

- Fourth degree burns cause extensive damage in the body and must receive medical care. They may injure nerves, blood vessels, muscles, tendons, ligaments, and bones.

Treating Thermal Burns

Burns sterilize the areas injured as well as the clothes worn in the affected area for a short period. Try to preserve their sterile nature for as long as possible.

Your main goal is to cool the skin down using cool, running water for 20 minutes, then assess the burn and the state of the distressed person. If no water is available. Follow the steps below.

1. Wash and sterilize your hands before assisting the person and handling the wound. Minimize handling of the wounded area.

2. Don't apply any lotions.

3. Don't remove clothing.

4. Don't break blisters.

5. Cover the affected area, including the burnt clothing, with a dry sterile dressing where possible. Clean lint or freshly laundered linen can also be used if no dressing is available.

6. When no blisters are present, bandage firmly. If blisters are present or suspected, bandage lightly.

7. Immobilize the affected area.

8. Treat the person for **shock**.

Treating Chemical Burns

Your priority: Flush out the chemical with a neutralizing agent and water.

For acids

1. Flush the affected area with water.

2. Bathe the affected area with copious amounts of an alkaline solution made from two teaspoons of baking soda or washing soda in one pint of warm water.

For Alkalis

1. If the burn is a result of quicklime, brush any residue off.

2. Bathe the affected area with copious amounts of a weak acid solution made from vinegar or lemon juice diluted in an equal amount of warm water.

Cuts and Wounds

Types of Cuts and Wounds

- **Incised wounds** are caused by sharp instruments such as a razor or metal vegetable peelers.

- **Lacerated wounds** are noted by their torn and irregular edges and are often caused by machinery, animal claws, kitchen graters, etc.

- **Contused wounds** are caused by a direct blow or crushing and are often accompanied by bruising in the affected area.

- **Puncture wounds** are caused by a stab from sharp, pointed instruments such as needles, knives, and bayonets. Though they may have quite small visible wounds, the instrument may penetrate quite deeply.

Treating Cuts and Wounds

Your priority: Reduce or stop bleeding, clean the wound, and pack or bandage the wound to prevent further opening of the wound.

1. Unless the person has a fracture, position them so that the wound is elevated.

2. Staunch the bleeding as much as possible before cleaning the wound. To stop the bleeding or staunch it, apply direct, steady pressure to the

elevated wound for a full 15 minutes. Use a clock or timer to ensure a full 15 minutes have passed before checking to see if bleeding is under control. Resist checking the wound before then. If blood fully saturates the cloth over the wound, add another cloth or gauze pad over the first one without disturbing it. If there's an object in the wound, don't apply direct pressure on the object; apply pressure around the object.

3. Don't disturb any blood clots that are forming.

4. Remove as little clothing as possible and expose the wound. Jewelry in the area of the wound should also be removed so that if swelling occurs, the jewelry doesn't impede blood flow.

5. Remove foreign bodies that can be easily wiped off with a clean dressing or which can be easily picked out without disturbing the wound.

6. Apply a clean bandage or dressing.

7. Immobilize the injury. If the injury is by a joint, use a splint if necessary.

Keep in Mind

- Mild bleeding usually stops or slows to a trickle after direct pressure is applied for 15 minutes. Sometimes, mild bleeding may still ooze for up to 45 minutes.

- If moderate to severe bleeding doesn't slow after 15 minutes of direct pressure, call for medical help while continuing to apply direct pressure to the wound.

- Don't use a tourniquet to stop bleeding.

- Clean the wound and do all you can to avoid further injury as well.

- If a foreign object is embedded in the wound and it cannot be easily removed, cover the object with a dressing. Stack sufficient pads around the wound without applying pressure to the object.

- If the cut is deep and there are no foreign objects present, ensure you pack padding into the wound's depths, and make sure you have sufficient pads at the skin level to apply pressure on ruptured blood vessels.

- While attending to the wound, monitor the person for **signs of shock**.

- Don't allow the person anything to eat or drink if their wound is severe as they may need an anesthetic. Moisten their lips with water if they are thirsty.

- While waiting for help, cover the person with a blanket if they are cold. Don't use a direct source of heat, such as a heat lamp to warm a severely wounded person.

Severed Finger or Toe

Severed fingers or toes can result from vehicles and machinery—workplaces or in the garden—or accidents involving knives and other sharp recreational equipment. A finger or toe can be reattached to a hand or foot if care is taken from the outset. In the event of a cut or wound involving a severed finger or toe, follow these steps:

1. If machinery or a vehicle is involved, turn it off.

2. Call emergency services or arrange transportation of the person to a trauma unit.

3. If others can assist, ask them to locate the appendage if it has been amputated, and follow the steps from 11-16. If there is no-one to help, locate the finger or toe after you have stopped the bleeding.

4. Without removing any clothing or jewelry from the injured hand or foot, elevate the injured limb.

5. Cleanse the wound with a saline solution.

6. Cover the injury with a sterile gauze or similar dressing.

7. Don't squeeze the wound or apply too much pressure on it as this causes further damage. Apply a light bandage if needed, and ensure circulation is good.

8. If the wound is still bleeding heavily, apply *light* pressure.

9. Treat the person for **shock**.

10. Don't allow the person any food or drink as they will be given an anesthetic at the hospital.

11. Once the amputated finger or toe is found, don't scrub it but wash it gently with a sterile saline solution.

12. Dampen a gauze dressing and wrap the appendage in it.

13. Place the finger or toe in a waterproof, clean, sealed plastic bag.

14. Into a larger plastic sealable bag, place the bag with the appendage.

15. Set the bundle on ice or surround it with ice or cold water in a cooler. Never place the severed finger or toe directly onto ice or cold water as this causes further damage.

16. If more than one finger or toe was severed right off, wrap them individually and seal in separate plastic bags to ensure the best outcome.

17. Ensure the severed appendages always travel with the person to the trauma unit so there is no delay in surgery.

Head Injuries

Most head injuries, from bumps to scrapes to cuts, are minor injuries that heal well with no professional medical care required. These minor injuries can be treated in the same way as we would bumps, scrapes, and cuts to other areas of the body. However, other head injuries can be life-threatening, from seemingly minor head bumps to concussion from contact sports.

Common Causes of Head Injuries

- Car crashes are responsible for almost half of adult head injuries, with young adults and teenagers most likely to sustain head injuries in car crashes.

- Falls in children under 5-years-old, and in older adults above 60.

- Sports and work-related accidents. Men have double the chance of sustaining head injuries than women at work and during sport. Many sports-related head injuries may not be reported.

- Violent attacks and assaults often result in head injuries, with gunshot wounds accounting for the leading cause of death from a head injury.

Signs of Head Injuries

- Severe facial or head bleeding

- Bleeding or fluid oozing from the ears and nose

- Vomiting

- Severe headache

- Change in consciousness that lasts more than a few seconds

- Black and blue discoloration below the eyes and behind the ears

- Not breathing

- Confusion

- Agitation

- Loss of balance

- Weakness or the inability to use limbs

- Unequal pupil size

- Slurred speech

- Blurred vision

In addition, children may also show these signs:

- Persistent crying

- Refusal to eat

- Bulging in the soft spot in front of the head in infants

- Repeated vomiting

Treating Head Injuries

Your priority: Keep their head and neck still. Stop the bleeding and assist with breathing if necessary.

1. Keep the person's head still.

2. Get them to lie down and elevate their shoulders. Avoid moving the person's neck or relocating them unless absolutely necessary. If they are wearing headgear such as a helmet, don't remove it.

3. Stop bleeding by applying direct pressure with sterile gauze or cloth unless you suspect a skull fracture.

4. Monitor the person for changes in breathing and alertness. If you find no breathing, heartbeat, coughing or other movement, begin CPR.

5. If the person is stable, look for signs or injury to other parts of the body and attend to them if needed.

Concussion

Concussion occurs when the brain comes into sharp contact with the inside of the skull from a blow to the head or a fall. Severe concussion can be dangerous if the person loses consciousness. It is vital to avoid sports and other activities that might result in a second concussion as a second impact can often lead to permanent brain damage or even be fatal if the first concussion is not fully healed. People may take between three months to a year to recover fully from a serious concussion.

Signs and Symptoms of Concussion

- Stare blankly (be dazed)

- Appear confused or cry for no reason

- Nausea

- Vomiting

- Headache

- Dizziness

- Memory loss (including amnesia)

- Blurry vision

- Ringing in the ears (tinnitus)

- Loss of taste and smell

- Irritability

- Slurred speech

- Sensitivity to light and noise.

When mild symptoms persist, medical care must be found.

Sometimes a person may experience post concussive syndrome for three months or even a year after the injury. Symptoms include blurred vision, forgetfulness, concentration problems, nausea, headache, and vomiting. Sometimes, there may be a change in personality, problems with balance and a lack of coordination, disruption of sleep patterns, depression and other psychological disorders, fatigue, and bouts of dizziness.

Assisting Someone Suffering from Concussion

Your priority: Monitor the person to determine if their symptoms are worsening and relay any information to medical professionals. If they have a severe concussion, it is best to wake them up gently every hour if medical help is delayed. If a child or infant shows signs of concussion, always get them swift medical care.

At home:

1. If you find the person's eyes are dilated (pupils are very large), they have difficulty walking and

maintaining their balance, or they can't hold a conversation, then wake them up every couple of hours and get them urgent medical attention.

2. If the person doesn't show the symptoms from 1., then it is safe and good for them to get as much rest as they need.

3. Ensure the person avoids sports and other heavy, physically demanding activities as well as driving.

4. Manage mentally demanding activities so they have less stress and more rest.

5. Recommend less exposure to electronic screens, including phones and avoiding alcohol and non-prescription drugs.

Poisoning

Poison is a toxic substance that makes a person feel sick or causes injuries to their mind and body. Over ninety percent of poisoning occurs at home. (Healthwise staff, 2018) Poisons are found in all households in the form of cleaning aids, houseplants, cosmetics, and even medication or supplements taken in the wrong dose or by someone who does not need the medication. Industrial chemicals are also toxic and can be found in homes and at work.

Poisons can cause harm when they are eaten, drunk, inhaled, in contact with your skin or your eyes. Products that give off fumes are generally considered poisonous, as are substances found in aerosol form.

Signs and Symptoms of Poisoning

Symptoms of poisoning can often be mistaken for seizures, strokes, insulin reaction, alcohol intoxication and other conditions.

Look for these signs and symptoms:

- Burns and redness around mouth and lips

- Breath that smells of chemicals such as paint thinner or gasoline

- Vomiting

- Difficulty breathing

- Drowsiness

- Confusion or other altered mental state

Treating Poisoning

Your priority: Identify the poison, remove contaminated clothing, assist in breathing, apply suitable steps to minimize harm from the identified poison. **Use a facemask or pocket mask if you are to give CPR.**

Note: Never induce vomiting in the person!

Stay calm and follow the steps below in order. Act as quickly as possible.

1. Check if the person is conscious.

2. Open the airway, ensuring their tongue isn't blocking their throat. Tilt their head back and lift their chin up with your forefinger and thumb while gently pressing their forehead back with your other hand. Position the person on their back. See **Opening The Airway** for more instructions.

3. Check if the person is breathing: look for the belly or chest moving up and down; feel the chest move up and down; feel the patient's breath on your cheek; put your ear close to the person's mouth and listen for sounds of their breathing.

4. If the person is not breathing after you've opened the airway, clear out the mouth and the throat. Turn their head to one side. Using one or two fingers, and preferably using gloves, scoop around the mouth and throat to clear out any vomit. Take care not to lodge any foreign objects down their throat. If the person wears false teeth, remove the dentures. If the person resumes breathing, turn them on their side into the recovery position. Check their pulse and breathing often. If the person doesn't resume breathing, you will need to help them breathe.

5. Give **mouth-to-mouth respiration** or mouth to nose respiration for an adult.

6. Check for a heartbeat. Feel for a pulse on the neck, in the hollow between the voice box and the muscle. Place two fingers on the Adam's Apple (voice box) and slide your fingers into the groove under the jaw. Feel for a pulse by holding your fingers in this position for at least five seconds. If the person has no pulse, they are in cardiac arrest. They will be unconscious, and their pupils will be large. Their skin will take on a blue-gray or ashen tinge or look for a blue tinge under their nails, to their lips, and the inside of their lower lids.

7. If they are in cardiac arrest, their breathing will also have stopped, and they will need both heart massage and mouth-to-mouth respiration. If their heart is beating, but they are not breathing, continue with mouth-to-mouth respiration. Take a deep breath and blow every five seconds until the person resumes breathing without help. You may need to do this for an hour. When the person starts to breathe, turn them onto their side and into the recovery position. The person may vomit when they resume breathing, but with them on their side, the vomit won't block their airway. Let the vomit drain out and then clear out their mouth with a finger.

8. If their heart is still not beating, give a heart massage.

How to Give a Heart Massage to an Adult

1. Check for a heartbeat. If there's none, commence with the heart massage.

2. On a firm surface, lay the person on their back. Kneel beside their chest.

3. Locate the right position to place your hands. From the lower edge of the ribs, follow the lower edge of the ribs to where they meet the breastbone. Place your middle finger at the base of the breastbone and your index finger next to it. Then place the heel of your other hand next to these two fingers, on the breastbone on the midline of the chest.

4. Cover your hand with your other hand and interlock your fingers so they are not touching the chest. Center your shoulders about the person's midline and straighten your arms.

5. Press down once on the lower half of the breastbone about four to five centimeters, keeping your arms straight. Then stop pressing. Count "And one and two and three" pressing down once for each count so you're doing 80 presses a

minute. Presses must be regular and smooth, not jabs.

6. Remember to give mouth-to-mouth resuscitation after every 15 presses. Tilt the head back to open the airway, seal your mouth over the person's mouth and give two breaths.

7. Continue with the two breaths for every 15 presses. After one minute, check for a heartbeat, then again after three minutes, then after every 12 cycles. As soon as the heartbeat resumes, stop the heart massage. The person's color may return to normal and their pupils may constrict.

8. Continue mouth-to-mouth respiration until the person breathes without help. It may take some time for breathing to resume even though the heart is now beating. When breathing resumes, position the person on their side in the recovery position. If you have another person to assist you, work as a team and get them to do the breathing while you do the heart massage.

9. If the person is unconscious, ensure they are in the recovery position.

10. Give first aid for **fits (convulsions)** if necessary.

11. Thoroughly wash any chemicals out of the person's eyes before washing the person's skin as any delay worsens the person's condition. Use lots of cool, clean water.

a. Gently brush or wipe off any powder, liquid, or residue from the person's face. Get the person to sit or lie down with their head tilted back and turned to the side worst affected. Open the person's affected eye (or eyes) and pour or run cold water over it, ensuring the water runs away from the person's body and doesn't cause any more harm. Though the person may be in great discomfort or pain, allowing them to keep their eyes closed will cause permanent damage. Gently, continue washing out the person's eye or eyes for 15 or 20 minutes, using a watch or a timer to ensure it is a full 15 to 20 minutes.

b. Ensure the inner lids are well rinsed. Ensure you've removed all solid pieces and residue of the chemical from between the folds of the eyes, the eyelashes, the eyebrows, and the hollows of the eyes. If you are not sure you've removed all traces of the chemical, then continue flushing out the eye for another 10 minutes.

c. Prevent the person from rubbing their eyes.

d. The person must be examined by a doctor as damage may be delayed.

e. If the person's eyes are sensitive to the light, cover the eye with a sterile eye pad or dry gauze pad. If no sterile pads are available, use a clean folded cloth.

f. Secure the pad with a bandage, but not too tightly, to help heal the eye.

12. Remove all contaminated clothing and wash the person's skin and hair.

a) Move the person to the nearest shower or suitable water source. If no water is available, gently wipe or dab the person's skin and hair with paper or cloth. Don't rub or scrub the person's skin.

b) Bathe the person's injury under cool or lukewarm running water, using a mild soap if available. If no running water is available, use buckets of water. Bathe the person as quickly as you can, using lots of water. Remember to protect yourself from the chemical. Use an apron and gloves if they are at hand. Avoid breathing in chemical fumes.

c) While bathing the person, remove any contaminated clothing, including that with vomit, and any shoes and wristwatches. It is important to work speedily. Cut out clothing contaminated by corrosive or highly poisonous substances.

d) If the person has multiple or large areas of contamination, wash them under a shower or use a hose. If necessary, remember to sluice their hair, in the groin, under their fingernails, and behind their ears. Continue to run water over the person for at least ten minutes. If you can still see chemicals on the person, or their skin feels soapy or sticky, continue washing them down until their skin feels normal. This may take up to an hour.

e) Ensure that all the water is draining away quickly and safely as it will be contaminated by the chemical.

f) Dry the person's skin gently with a clean, soft towel. If clothing remains stuck to their skin even after bathing them, don't attempt to remove the cloth.

g) As poisons can seep through skin quickly, look for signs of poisoning.

h) Put contaminated clothes in a separate sealed container. Wash thoroughly before use. Throw out shoes that are contaminated. If cloth and paper were used to wash the person, put them in a sealed container and burn them.

13. Give first aid for poisonous **bites and stings.**

Heat Stroke

When a person's body temperature rises quickly and they can't cool themselves sufficiently, heat stroke occurs. A person can easily be overcome by heat stroke without being aware of it by staying in a hot environment for too long or by undertaking strenuous activity in the heat. Heat stroke is dangerous as it causes damage to a person's brain and other vital organs. Children and animals (particularly those left in cars) are very susceptible to heat stroke, as are the elderly.

Signs and Symptoms

- Fever of 104 F (40 C) or higher

- Changes in behavior such as slurred speech, agitation, or confusion

- Hot, dry skin or heavy sweating

- Nausea and vomiting

- Flushed skin

- Rapid pulse

- Rapid breathing

- Headache

- Fainting (usually the first sign in older adults)

Treating Heat Stroke

Your priority: Move the person out of the heat and cool their bodies down as quickly as possible, then hydrate the person.

1. Quickly move the person out of the heat.

2. Remove restrictive and heavy clothing.

3. Cool them in the best way you can including:

a) Place the person under a cool shower or in a cool tub.

b) Spray with a garden hose.

c) Sponge with cold water.

d) Fan while misting with cold water.

e) Place ice packs, wet towels, or cold compresses under the armpits, groin and neck.

f) Cover with cool, damp sheets.

4. Feed the person cool water to rehydrate.

5. Don't allow the person sugary, caffeinated, or alcoholic drinks. Cold and icy beverages should also be avoided as they will cause stomach cramps.

6. Begin CPR if the person stops breathing and loses consciousness, showing no sign or circulation, coughing or other movement.

Hypothermia and Frostbite

Hypothermia

When your body loses heat faster than it can produce it, and your temperature drops below 95 F (35 C), you experience hypothermia. Untreated hypothermia quickly becomes life-threatening.

Hypothermia occurs when a person has prolonged exposure to cold in any season; from cold weather to immersion in cold water to exposure to indoor cooling below 50 F (10 C). The risk of hypothermia is increased by exhaustion and dehydration.

Signs and Symptoms of Hypothermia

Symptoms of hypothermia develop gradually and may include:

- Shivering, which may stop as the condition worsens and the person's body temperature drops

- Slurred speech or mumbling

- Slow, shallow breathing

- Weakness

- Clumsiness of lack of coordination

- Drowsiness or low energy

- Confusion or memory loss

- Loss of consciousness

- Bright red, cold skin (in infants)

What Not to Do in the Event of Hypothermia

- Don't rapidly warm the person up with a heating lamp or hot bath.

- Don't attempt to warm the arms and legs of the person as this may stress their heart.

- Don't give the person cigarettes or alcohol. Alcohol complicates the body's heating process and can exacerbate the situation. Cigarettes hinder circulation that is required to help the person recover.

Treating Hypothermia

Your priority: Keep the person from further cold, raise their core temperature gradually without rubbing their limbs.

1. Move the person out of the cold as gently as possible.

2. If there is no shelter, shield the person from the wind, particularly their head and neck. Insulate them from the cold ground.

3. Gently remove wet clothing. Replace with dry, warm coats and blankets.

4. If more warmth is required, apply it gradually. For example, help heat the person's core by applying hot compresses to the torso of the body—neck, chest and groin. The CDC recommends using an electric blanket, if available. If you are using heat packs or hot water bottles, wrap them in towels first.

5. Feed the person warm, sweet, non-alcoholic drinks.

6. Begin CPR if the person slips into unconsciousness and shows no signs of life—no sign of breathing, coughing or movement.

Frostbites Vs Hypothermia

Frostbite occurs when your skin freezes during exposure to cold weather or water. It is common and often underestimated during winter fun activities but can still cause damage to your body.

While hypothermia is more serious and affects your body as a whole, frostbite, though localized, damages skin cells and tissue in the exposed parts of your skin by freezing them. Children, the elderly, people with hypertension or diabetes, smokers, alcohol consumers, and drug users are most at risk from frostbite.

Symptoms of frostbite include feelings of "pins and needles," numbness, swelling, blisters, loss of coordination and blackened skin.

While frostbite might seem less severe than hypothermia, the long-term effects of untreated and repeated frostbite are costly. Nerves may be damaged, affecting your sensitivity, while frostbite arthritis may affect you years later. Frostbite arthritis causes swelling and stiffness of your joints.

Prevention of Frostbite

Dress according to the weather with layers and windproof and waterproof gear. Ensure your fingers and toes are protected. Avoid recreational drugs, alcohol, and heavy exercise when in icy winds. Ensure you are hydrating. Go out in the cold only if necessary and keep trips short. Ensure your clothing and shoes don't cut off your circulation.

Treating Frostbite

Your priority: Remove wet clothing, gently warm skin with warm water.

Self-treatment:

1. Prioritize staying warm and preventing freezing again to avoid further skin damage.

2. To warm up:

a. Remove any wet clothing.

b. Elevate the frostbitten area slightly. Don't rub frostbitten areas as this can cause tissue damage.

c. Warm your skin by soaking in warm water that is about 105 F (40.5 C). Don't use heat sources to warm your skin such as heaters, fires, or electric blankets.

d. Be careful not to burn the area with hot water as the skin will be numb and burning the area will cause more damage to your skin. Once your fingers are soft again, remove them from the warm water.

e. Cover the frostbitten area with a sterile (clean) cloth. If your fingers or toes were affected, ensure they are wrapped individually to avoid stress and pressure to them.

f. Try to keep the area affected immobile. Don't walk with frostbitten feet.

Fractures

Bones are often fractured in accidents and falls. When there's no wound on the skin, it's a simple fracture.

General Symptoms and Signs of Fracture

- Pain at or near the point of the fracture

- Discomfort and tenderness when pressure is applied over the area of the fracture

- Swelling in the affected area may make it difficult to identify or assess the extent of the fracture. Take care to detect other signs of fracture.

- Deformity of the limb

- Irregularity of the bone

Treating Fractures

Your priority: Stop the bleeding if there is any and immobilize the limb with a splint.

Set your priorities.

1. Treat the fracture immediately. Unless in a life-threatening environment, don't move the person until the fractured limb has been immobilized. If necessary, immobilize the limb temporarily, then move the person as short a distance as possible to a safer area where a sturdier fix can be done.

2. Bleeding and open wounds must be attended to first, before the setting of the fracture.

3. Steady and support the injured area first, ensuring the person cannot bend or move the limb. This prevents further injury and bleeding, as well as minimizes the risk of broken splinters of

bone causing internal injury to muscle, skin, nerves, and blood vessels.

4. **Splint the limb** with bandages or other suitable items so the limb is completely immobilized.

Electrocution

When a person touches a live or naked wire, cable or rail, the shock experienced can range from mild to severe. In the case of severe shock, a burn will result. In the case of high voltages, burns may be severe or deep.

A live current passing through a person's body can be life-threatening and result in cardiac arrest and other injuries. Any electrocution can be fatal; a high voltage is not necessary.

When a shock has occurred, swift action can save a person's life.

Treating Electrocution

If the person is still in contact with the electric current, do not touch them.

Your priority: Remove the source of the current from the person and, if it's safe for you to do so, assist the person with breathing and circulation.

1. Switch off the current or cut off the supply by unplugging the source of the shock, wrenching it

free or breaking the cable, taking care not to touch the live end yourself. If that's not possible, move the source away from you and the person with a non-conductive, dry object made from cardboard, plastic, or wood. Never use metal or attempt to cut a cable with a knife or scissors.

2. With utmost care, remove the person from contact with the current using dry, insulated materials. At home, use a folded garment, gloves, or newspaper for protection.

3. Reassure the patient.

4. Lay the person on their back with their head positioned so that it is low and turned to one side unless they are injured on their head, chest or abdomen; then raise their head and shoulders slightly and ensure their head is supported.

5. Loosen clothing around their neck, chest, and waist.

6. Do not give the person any fluids until the paramedics arrive.

7. Begin CPR if the person isn't breathing, has no heartbeat, or otherwise shows no signs of circulation.

8. Keep the person from getting chilled.

9. Apply a sterile gauze bandage or a clean cloth to any burn areas. Never use a towel or a blanket as the loose fibers can stick to the burns.

Clothes on Fire

Fire is a common urgency that is horrifying in its ability to cause us to panic and to escalate into a disaster. If a person's clothes catch fire, use the Stop, Drop, Roll method then ensure the fire is under control.

Helping Someone with Their Clothes on Fire

Your priority: Roll the person (if they have no neck, head, or spinal injury) on the floor to snuff out the fire.

1. Stop. Reassure the person and talk to them calmly through the next two steps. If they are panicking, be firm and do the actions with them.

2. Drop. Drop to the ground as swiftly as possible. Cover them with a non-flammable coat, rug, or fire blanket if possible.

3. Roll immediately. Help the person roll their body. This should snuff out the fire on their clothes.

4. Assess any burns.

5. Call emergency services.

6. **Treat any burns** until help arrives.

Difficulty in Swimming or Drowning

Children, pets, and the elderly can often fall into water or experience difficulty while swimming in water.

Your priority: Help them out of the water only if it is safe for you to do so. Prevent water from damaging lungs and brain. Assist in breathing if necessary and keep them warm. Get the person to a medical facility to prevent secondary drowning—when air passages swell hours after lungs are affected by immersion in water.

Helping Someone Immersed in Water or Drowning

1. Don't get into the water if you are not a trained lifesaver. Dial emergency services or call for help.

2. If it is safe to do so, hold out a hand, a stick, or throw a floating object.

3. Assist the person out of the water, ensuring you don't fall in yourself.

4. Keep them warm.

5. Set them in the recovery position, preferably with their head lower than the rest of their body so they can't inhale any more water.

6. Ensure their airways are clear.

7. Remove wet clothing if dry clothes are available and treat them for **hypothermia**.

8. Arrange for transport to a medical facility with a doctor.

Caring for Someone in Isolation or Quarantine at Home

Only one adult should care for the person or come into any contact with them. If this adult is you, ensure that should you be sick, another elected able adult or the oldest teenager can take over your duties and knows whom to contact for help. Ensure the stand-by carer is not pregnant.

Your priority: Tend to the isolating person's daily needs with food, water, medication and any other help they may require. Avoid the infection yourself. Monitor the person for aggravated symptoms of the infection.

Points to Remember

- Keep the isolating person away from others in the home. The isolating person should stay in a bedroom with the door closed, and preferably, if possible, have a bathroom for their own use only.

- Don't allow any visitors.

- Keep pets away from the isolating person as pets can become infected by certain diseases, too. Also, it is harder and more traumatic to disinfect pets regularly than it is for people.

- Keep all items used by the isolating person separate from those of the general household. This includes bedding and linen, toiletries, cutlery, mugs, and dinnerware, and unwashed clothes. Handle the isolating person's laundry with gloves or plastic bags on your hands.

- Ensure the isolating person rests and is well nourished.

- Encourage the isolating person to exercise if they are well enough to do so.

- When interacting with other people, for example in the garden or other common areas, wear a well-fitted mask and stay at least 1.5 meters (5 ft) away.

- Always disinfect the area the isolating person has been in with a reputable disinfectant.

- Wash your hands often.

- Monitor the isolating person for any further symptoms or deterioration of their condition. If they do produce symptoms or their condition worsens, get medical help.

- If you have applied first aid to an isolating person, take extra precautions with wound treatment and CPR, and ensure all waste is specially marked and incinerated at a suitable facility.

- If you've called for medical help for a person in isolation, let the dispatchers know that the person in distress is isolating.

As for the rest of the household:

- Maintain a positive attitude.

- Discuss the infection openly and ensure everyone is informed about the health of the person in quarantine.

- Keep the household routine as normal as possible.

- Exercise regularly, outdoors if possible, to alleviate stress and depression.

- Maintain contact with family and friends via conference calling or messaging.

- Remember quarantines usually end after a two-week period and that you and your family have the resilience to cope.

CHAPTER 5:

RESPONDING TO EMERGENCIES RELATED TO PERMANENT MEDICAL CONDITIONS

A person with a permanent medical condition can sometimes find themselves in an emergency medical situation resulting from their chronic illness. We will look at how to deal with some of the more common emergencies resulting from chronic health conditions such as epileptic seizures, heart attacks, and severe allergic reactions.

Heart Attacks and Chest Pains

Heart attacks occur when the flow of blood to the heart is blocked. Blockages may be caused by blood clots, blood plaque (cholesterol) in arteries, or collapsed blood vessels. Treatment during the first 90 minutes of an attack greatly increases the chance the person's life will be saved.

While not all chest pains are a sign of heart attack, it usually denotes a medical condition and you should ensure that the person gets medical attention.

Symptoms for Both Genders

- Discomfort and pain in the chest area; or a feeling of pressure, tightness, or an aching and squeezing sensation at the center of the chest for more than 15 minutes.

- Pain that spreads to the shoulders, arms, neck, back, jaw, teeth, and sometimes the abdomen.

- Indigestion, heartburn, nausea, vomiting, or abdominal pain

- Shortness of breath

- Dizziness, fainting, light-headedness

- Sweating

- A racing or irregular heartbeat

Specific Symptoms for Men

Most men experience cold sweats while pain may travel down their left arm.

Specific Symptoms for Women

Women tend to have more indistinct symptoms such as nausea, stomach upsets, dizziness, tiredness, shortness of breath, jaw, or back pain.

Treating Heart Attacks

1. If the medication is available, give the person an aspirin, or if they have a doctor's prescription for nitroglycerin, then ensure they take the correct dosage at once. Aspirin reduces the incidences of blood clots and reduces damage to the heart if the person is experiencing a heart attack.

2. If you don't have access to medication and the person is unconscious, is not breathing and you find no pulse, begin **CPR**. Press hard and fast in a rapid rhythm of 100 to 120 presses a minute.

Stroke

When a blood vessel in the brain bursts or is blocked, a person has a stroke. With its oxygen and blood cut off, the affected part of the brain begins to die, and the body functions that part of the brain controls are not available to the person. For instance, they may not be able to speak if their speech centers are affected.

It is important to know the signs of stroke and to act fast as brain damage can occur within minutes of the stroke. Receiving medical help quickly not only reduces brain damage, but also makes a full recovery possible.

Signs of a Stroke

- Sudden weakness, numbness, tingling or loss of movement in the face, arm, or leg, particularly on one side of the body.

- Sudden vision loss in one eye: blurred vision, dim vision, or no vision

- Sudden speech problems

- Sudden confusion and no understanding of even simple statements

- Sudden problems with movement or balance; loss of bowel and bladder control

- Sudden severe headache unlike those usually experienced

- Quite often, most strokes are painless.

FAST is a simple way to remember the symptoms of stroke:

- F - face drooping

- A - arm weakness

- S - Speech difficulty

- T - Time to call 911

Treating Stroke Victims

1. Ensure they are in a safe, comfortable position and environment. Lay them on their side with their head supported in case they vomit.

2. Check their breathing. If they stop breathing, administer **CPR**. If they're having trouble breathing, loosen tight clothing such as ties and scarves.

3. Reassure them by talking to them in a calm tone.

4. Keep them warm. Cover them with a blanket.

5. If they are weak, particularly in a limb, don't move them.

6. Observe the person for a change in their condition. Be prepared to tell emergency operators and responders the person's symptoms and when they first appeared. If the person fell and hit their head, mention that as soon as possible.

7. Perform CPR as needed.

8. Stay calm and alert.

What Not to Do in the Case of Stroke

- Don't allow the person any drink or food.

- Don't drive to the hospital. Wait for emergency services.

- Don't give the person any medication.

- The key to stroke treatment is getting hospital treatment as soon as possible. Patients taken to hospital in an ambulance get diagnosed and are treated much quicker than a patient not arriving in an ambulance.

Seizures

Seizures may be caused by epilepsy, as a reaction to incorrect medication, or other medical or traumatic reasons.

Signs and Symptoms

- Loss of consciousness

- Muscle contractions and convulsions

- Weakness

- Clouded awareness

- Loss of sensation

- Fidgeting

- Strange sensations in the stomach

- Confusion and sleepiness after the seizure

In the Event of a Seizure

Your aim is to keep the person safe until the seizure stops.

1. Loosen any clothing around the person's neck.

2. Lay them on the floor.

3. Don't attempt to restrain them or put any objects in their mouth.

4. Clear the area and ensure there are no hard objects nearby.

5. Stay with them until the seizure stops.

Severe Allergic Reactions or Anaphylaxis

A severe allergic reaction (anaphylaxis) can be life-threatening as it may cause a shock, a sudden drop in blood pressure, or interfere with breathing.

People with allergies may experience reactions minutes after exposure to the allergen. Sometimes there can be a delay before anaphylaxis occurs, or even no apparent trigger.

Signs and Symptoms

- Skin reactions including rashes, paleness, red skin, itching or hives

- Swelling on the face, lips, eyes, or throat.

- Constriction of the throat with wheezing or trouble breathing

- A weak and rapid pulse

- Diarrhea, nausea, vomiting

- Dizziness, fainting or losing consciousness.

Treating a Person with a Severe Allergic Reaction

Your aim is to help the person use their allergy medication, assist them with breathing if necessary, and get them to a medical care facility.

1. Ask the person if they are carrying an epinephrine auto injector (Epipen, Auvi-Q,or others) to treat an allergy attack.

2. If the person has an auto injector, ask them whether you should help them inject the medication. This is usually done by pressing the auto injector against the person's thigh.

3. Lay the person down on their back. Keep them still.

4. Loosen tight clothing and cover the person with a blanket. Don't give them anything to drink.

5. If they are vomiting or bleeding from the mouth, turn them to their side so the fluids can drain and they won't choke.

6. If the person stops breathing and shows no signs of coughing or other movement, begin CPR. Do uninterrupted compressions of about 100 every minute until paramedics arrive.

7. Get the person emergency medical treatment. After anaphylaxis, monitoring at a hospital is usually necessary as symptoms can reoccur.

What Not to Do

- Don't delay treatment by waiting to see if symptoms improve. Seek immediate emergency treatment. In severe cases, death can result within half an hour.

- An antihistamine pill isn't a sufficient treatment for anaphylaxis. While they may relieve symptoms, they can't fight off the damage a severe allergic reaction does to the body.

Asthma

Asthma is so prevalent that every ten seconds someone in the world is having a potentially life-threatening attack. (NHS Choices. 2019) Their chances of having a severe attack is greatly reduced if they are on the right treatment.

Signs and Symptoms

Take action when the follow signs and symptoms worsen:

- Coughing, wheezing, tightness in their chest, or breathlessness

- Their usual reliever or inhaler isn't helping

- Feeling too breathless to talk, eat, or sleep

- Breathing rate is going up and they still cannot catch their breath

- The person's peak flow score is lower than normal

- Children, in addition, may complain of chest or stomach ache.

Treating an Asthma Attack

1. Sit the person upright (not lying down), and coach them to take slow, steady breaths.

2. Reassure them and help them remain calm as panicking will worsen their condition.

3. Encourage them to take long, deep breaths. This helps to prevent hyperventilation by slowing down their breathing. Have them breathe in through their nose and out through their mouth.

4. Help them move away from the trigger and into clean air or an air-conditioned place. The asthma attack could be triggered by dust, cigarette smoke, or the smell of chemicals such as ammonia, chlorine gas or sulfur dioxide.

5. Give them a hot caffeinated beverage. This may help open their airways a little and provide relief for a short while.

6. Let them take one puff of their usual inhaler every 30 to 60 seconds for a maximum of 10 puffs.

7. Repeat every 15 minutes.

8. If their condition improves, they don't require emergency medical care, but they do need to consult their doctor as soon as possible.

Tachycardia or Heart Palpitations

Heart palpitations occur when the person feels as if their heart is pounding, or fluttering, at an alarmingly high rate.

These palpitations may last for a few seconds and may occur at any time.

While not all palpitations are caused by a heart condition, they can be caused by other factors that put stress on your heart, such as illness, dehydration, general stress, exercise, caffeine, pregnancy, illegal drugs, or tobacco products.

Treating Heart Palpitations

In most cases, no treatment is needed. You can help alleviate the person's condition by:

1. Trying relaxation techniques.

2. Giving them water to drink water.

3. Encouraging them to do vagal maneuvers.

4. Encouraging them to avoid stimulants.

5. Restoring electrolyte balance.

Hyperglycemia

One of the two conditions resulting from diabetes, hyperglycemia occurs in any age group when a person with Type 1 diabetes runs out of insulin. As their bodies don't produce insulin, they are dependent on their insulin injections, pumps, and injection pen.

Hyperglycemia develops slowly over a few hours or days and often leads to a diabetic coma which must be treated in hospital.

Signs of Hyperglycemia

- Sweet breath with a fruity smell

- Hyperventilation or rapid breathing and pulse

- Drowsiness

- Warm, dry skin.

While you can't treat a diabetic coma and hyperglycemia, **your priority** is to call for immediate medical care and to monitor the person. If they lose consciousness and stop breathing, give them CPR until medical help arrives.

Hypoglycemia

The second condition resulting from diabetes known as Type 2 hypoglycemia usually occurs in mature people or those suffering from obesity. As their body's sugar and insulin shifts out of balance, they become distressed and more ill.

Hyperglycemia develops fast if a meal is skipped or the person has exerted themselves too much. This condition often occurs in recently diagnosed diabetics who are still adjusting to their insulin regime and new lifestyle.

Signs of Hypoglycemia

- Weakness, faintness, or hunger.

- Muscle tremors

- Weak pulse

- Palpitations

- Cold clammy skin

- Sweating

- Confusion, irritability, or irrationality

- The person may be aware of their condition and history of diabetes and carry medication or wear a bracelet

- Responses grow erratic

Treating Hypoglycemia

Your priority: Raising the blood-sugar level of the person as fast as possible, then finding medical care.

1. Sit the person down as soon as possible.

2. If the person is carrying sugar, glucose, or candy, help them ingest them. If the person has no sugar products on them, give them two teaspoons of

sugar, a hard sugar candy, or a cup of regular soda (not the diet variants), or fruit juice.

3. If the person is recovering well, feed them more food and drink and allow them to rest.

4. Once they're feeling much better, help them do their glucose test if they carry a personal kit, or to find medical help.

5. Monitor the person.

6. If the person doesn't respond well to sugar intake, look for other conditions for their distress and stay with them until professional medical care arrives.

Chapter 6:

Alternative Medicine for

Emergencies

You may not always have your medical kit at hand, but you may have your larder or other resources available that may help in an emergency. Alternative and herbal remedies have been used in emergency situations for centuries. We'll look at some of the alternative herbal remedies the Red Cross of America and others recommend for your first aid kit.

Disclaimer

Natural remedies are extremely potent, interact with medications in unpredictable ways, and can be toxic and lead to poisoning or exacerbation of symptoms. If a person is allergic to any ingredient of a natural remedy, do not give it to them. Therefore, all homemade natural remedies must be precisely labeled with the ingredients (including carrier oils, alcohols, or other carrier and preserving agents), the date made, the expected expiration date, and dosage or instructions for use. These labels must be in indelible or waterproof ink.

Herbal remedies should be administered with great care or not at all (depending on the herb) to pregnant women, infants, young children, diabetics, people with high blood pressure, and people with existing kidney or liver conditions.

Herbs and spice-based remedies build up concentrations in your body the more often you take them. If taken over extended periods of time, this can lead to toxicity and illness. Therefore, herbal remedies should be taken in small doses (some even minuscule), and immune boosters and other supplements and preventative remedies should be taken on an on-and-off basis to allow concentrations to deplete safely.

If a person experiences an allergic reaction to an initial dose or other negative reaction, the preparation should no longer be used to treat them.

If you have been using herbal supplements to treat someone, inform any medical professional who takes over attending the ill or distressed person.

Notes for Storing Natural Remedies in First Aid Kits

- Store ingredients in airtight containers.

- Wrap glass bottles in paper or cloth to prevent leakage and cushion them. Label on the outside.

- Ensure all ingredients, instructions for use, and dates are noted on the containers.

- Check powders regularly to ensure they are moisture-free.

- If an ointment, salve, cream smells 'off' or rancid, don't use it.

Manuka Honey

Manuka honey usually doesn't spoil and can be kept safely in your first aid kit for long periods of time.

Use Manuka Honey for:

- **Burns**. Manuka honey is now widely accepted as an excellent treatment for burns and wounds. Even conventional medical care is using manuka honey in burn treatment as it has natural antiseptic properties and prevents bacteria and viruses from entering wounds.

- **Sore throats**. Slowly suck a teaspoon to relieve a sore throat.

- **Energy boost**. Eat the honey for a quick energy boost or for much-needed calories.

Manuka Oil

Manuka oil has been shown to kill viruses (antiviral), bacteria (antibacterial), and fungi (antifungal).

Use Manuka Oil for:

- **Skin abrasions**

- Abscesses, blisters, bedsores, boils, sores

- Tonsillitis, ulcers, varicose veins

- Cold sores, acne, carbuncles, pimples

- Cracked skin, dermatitis, eczema

- Dandruff, fungal infections, lice, ringworm

- Infections from body piercings, insect bites, nail infections

- Rhinitis, sunburn, oily skin, tinea

Colloidal Silver

Colloidal Silver is similar to Manuka in that it is used to **prevent infections in wounds**. It may **treat food poisoning** when taken in safe doses internally. It may also help **manage eye infections** with a few drops in the eye before bed. It has been known to also help with ear infections and to help alleviate stomach bugs. However, Colloidal Silver must be taken in the correct dosage if used internally as it may have side effects depending on the distillation.

Live Aloe Vera

Clear sap from an aloe plant has similar wound healing and antibacterial uses as Manuka. As a broken leaf of the plant seals itself, you can carry the leaf with you.

Use Live Aloe Vera to:

- Apply directly to burns, cuts, and scrapes.

- Alleviate sunburn.

- Pack it in a flesh wound until medical help arrives.

Taken internally, aloe vera is believed to help relieve intestinal issues.

Cayenne Pepper

Taken internally, cayenne pepper acts as a vasodilator, opening up blood vessels. It can be used for emergency stroke treatment, heart attacks, and is often used in conjunction with other herbs to deliver the properties of the other herbs via the bloodstream to the area needing treatment.

It is also believed to aid sluggish circulation by applying it to the skin or soaking feet in warm water with some cayenne pepper in it.

Cayenne pepper also works well as a muscle relaxant, either taken internally, or if applied topically with a cream.

Black or Green Tea Bags

Black and green tea bags, or any caffeinated tea bag with large amounts of tannin, can be used to help stop bleeding. Wrap the wet tea bag in gauze and bite down on it to stop dental bleeding, or hold it against the wound, or secure it with a bandage on limbs and other areas of the body. (McDermott & Sullivan, 2017).

Green tea bags can also be used as a compress on eyes for conjunctivitis (place it on the eye for about 15 to 20 minutes), with the green tea being used as an eyewash. Green tea bags can also be used as a cold compress on skin irritations.

Chamomile

Chamomile is anti-inflammatory and relaxes the body. Chamomile tea or salves can work as muscle relaxants and provide relief from skin irritation, sore muscles, and anxiety. Inhaling steam from an infusion of chamomile flowers or tea also helps provide relief from sinus congestion. Take care not to burn your skin with the steam.

Arnica Gel or Cream

Arnica flowers improve circulation and have antibacterial properties.

To Use Arnica Gel or Cream:

- Apply it to sprain, strains, sore muscles.

- Apply it to bumps and bruises to reduce swelling.

- Taken internally as a liquid or homeopathic preparation, it can help relieve headaches and help tissues heal after surgery.

Calendula Cream

Calendula cream is made from *Calendula Officinalis*, also known as marigolds. Use it to treat scrapes, cuts, bruises, and open sores. It can be used if no antibacterial or antiseptic wash is available.

Rescue Remedy

Made from five Bach flower remedies, Rescue Remedy helps *you* stay calm when dealing with emergencies. Use it when dealing with physical shock and to keep you focused on following the steps to help a person in distress.

Rubbing Alcohol and Hydrogen Peroxide

Both Rubbing Alcohol and Hydrogen Peroxide have very long shelf-lives and are very affordable.

Use Rubbing Alcohol and Hydrogen Peroxide to:

- Clean light wounds when water and soap aren't available.

- Treat colds and flu by dropping a **3% solution of hydrogen peroxide** into the ear. However, if the person has an ear infection or a perforated eardrum, this is not recommended.

Ginger

Ginger has long been used in the East for its strong anti-inflammatory, antimicrobial and digestive properties. Use a piece of fresh ginger about the size of your fingernail. Alternatively, allow the person to drink up to two cups of ginger a day as larger quantities of ginger can cause stomach irritation.

Use Ginger to:

- Settle an upset stomach

- Aid with digestion

- Relieve abdominal gas and cramping

- Treat bacteria-induced diarrhea

- Alleviate symptoms of food poisoning

- Fight viral infections such as colds and relieve some of the symptoms

- Help dissolve mucus congestion and to induce sweating to overcome a cold fever, or flu

- Relieve nausea and vomiting

- Relieve motion sickness.

- Relieve morning sickness. **However, great caution must be used as ginger in larger amounts can affect pregnancy.**

- Relieve a sore throat, coughing, post-nasal drip, and mucus congestion as it is a natural analgesic

- Relieve the pain and swelling from rheumatoid arthritis, gout, and osteoarthritis

- Relieve menstrual pain and cramps. **Caution must be used as ginger may promote bleeding.**

- Provide relief from migraine pain, nausea, and dizziness as it can act as a pain blocker and reduce inflammation

- Lower cholesterol levels, blood pressure, and prevent blood clots so the risk of heart disease is reduced

- Fight allergic reaction, reduce asthma attacks, fight inflammation of the airways and fight respiratory viruses

Activated Charcoal or Bentonite Clay

Activated charcoal and bentonite clay both work to reduce toxins and poisons, so are helpful in overcoming food poisoning and stomach upsets.

Mix it into a paste and apply it to insect bites and stings to remove the toxins.

Activated charcoal can also be used to filter water in remote locations if water of drinking quality is scarce or unavailable.

Echinacea and Elderberry

Echinacea and elderberry are immune-boosting herbs that may shorten the duration of colds and the flu. Take at the first hint of exposure.

Eucalyptus

Eucalyptus oil is a natural antibiotic and antiviral. Mix a few drops of the essential oil in a carrier oil such as olive oil or coconut oil and use a vapor rub.

Use eucalyptus to:

- Help open congested airways

- Treat colds

- Treat sinus problems

- Support treatment of respiratory problems

Lavender

Lavender essential oil is often used to soothe and calm. Mix in a carrier oil before use.

Use Lavender to:

- Relieve headaches by rubbing onto the temples

- Reduce anxiety

- Treat insomnia

- Apply over the chest or over the feet for soothing relief

Tea Tree Oil

Tea Tree oil is a natural antiseptic.

Use Tea Tree Oil to:

- Treat bacterial infections as an alternative to antibacterial cream

- Prevent infections

- Heal cuts and bruises

- Treat minor skin burns

- Repel fungal problems such as athlete's foot and infected toenails.

- Relieve discomfort from insect bites

Witch Hazel

Witch Hazel is an astringent, antiseptic, and anti-inflammatory and is often used as a skin tonic and deodorant.

Use Witch Hazel to:

- Treat skin irritations such as rashes and insect bites

- Mix or dilute essential oils by using it as a carrier base

Acupuncture and Acupressure

Acupuncture is the application of pressure or needles to special points in the body. It has been proven as an effective means of pain relief and is used extensively in the UK and Germany in conventional medical centers as part of pain management treatments.

NB! If you are not trained in acupressure, acupuncture, or massage, don't press too hard on these points. If the person experiences a high level of discomfort or is further distressed by acupressure, then switch to another treatment.

Don't use acupressure or acupuncture on a pregnant woman as this can induce contractions.

Treatments with Acupuncture and Acupressure

To apply acupuncture to a point in the body, press down with one or two fingers at the point for about a minute. The correct point to treat will feel harder or be sore to the person being treated.

- **For headaches:** Between the thumb and forefinger, pinch the web of flesh.

- **For nausea:** Place three fingers on the wrist. At the point of the forearm next to the third finger, depress the crease or slight hollow just off-center for about a minute.

- **For neck pain and migraines:** Press the hollows at the back of the base of your skull.

- **For heartburn and indigestion:** Measure six finger widths from your navel and two below the end of your rib cage. Depress the middle of your torso at that point.

- **For nosebleeds:** Wrap twine, a ribbon, or a shoelace around the width of the palm. Ask the person to make a fist with that palm for about a minute to activate all the pressure points.

Artemisia Annua

In combination with other medical preparations, this Chinese herb is now considered among the most effective treatments for malaria. Used in China since the 3rd century, the herb is now available in a tablet form for oral use.

Recipes for First Aid Material

Sometimes, you may run out of salves, creams, and ointments to treat minor emergencies, burns, and stings and running to the pharmacy is not an option. Fortunately, you can make your own salves, creams, and ointments at home with a few ingredients. Remember to label your DIY first aid essentials with instructions and expiration date.

Next, you'll find some basic recipes to create a base for your cream, ointment, or salve. Variations will follow to help you create your own must-have soothing and antiseptic applications.

NB! Before using any of your own herbal creations, be sure to do a patch test to ensure it is safe to use. Discard immediately any batches that may be contaminated by other ingredients, or preparations that develop mold as they could cause infections or become poisonous.

Essential oils are not recommended for use by infants and pregnant women. Children and sensitive individuals should use essential oils sparingly except for lavender and rose.

How to Make Your Own Herbal Remedies

Basic Equipment

- clean glass jars with metal lids, metal containers, or glass bottles that seal well (Boil them in water to sterile them if you've used them before)

- wooden spatula or spoon

- wooden chopsticks or stirrers

- sauce pot

- double boiler

- mesh strainer

- muslin cloth, cheesecloth, or coffee/oil filters

- parchment paper (optional) or paper sandwich bags

- blender

- wooden, stone, or ceramic blending bowl

- tinted glass bottles

- droppers

Basic Ingredients

- beeswax

- carrier oils such as olive oil, sweet almond oil, coconut oil, jojoba oil, or grapeseed oil (you can blend different ones to make one that suits your needs)

- essential oils of your choice

- dried herbs as per your choice

- raw honey

- water (distilled)

- infused oils (you can make your own or buy them)

- witch hazel water

- aloe vera

- vodka or grain alcohol 40-50% alcohol (80-90 proof)

- vodka or grain alcohol 70-100% alcohol

- fresh herbs

- glycerin (glycerol)

- apple cider vinegar

Note: Before you make your own herbal preparations

Always do research and take notes for your preparation labels about each herb or ingredient regarding who can take it safely, and any other precautions or warnings. This is because each herb has different properties and so interacts with a person's body chemistry and medication in a different way. It is especially important to note if the herb or spice interacts with common medications and chronic health conditions such as diabetes, high blood pressure, people on blood thinners, etc.

Also, take into consideration that experimenting with different mixtures of herbs causes chemical reactions, which may give you very different properties or even produce poisonous results. Unless you are trained in herbology, it's best to stick to well-known and trusted combinations and quantities.

Basic Salve Recipe

This salve should keep for up to one year.

1. ½ cup of two base oils or 1 cup of oil. (8 Oz). Warm your base oils (coconut, olive, jojoba, grapeseed, etc.) in a saucepan or double boiler on medium heat.

2. ¼ cup each dried herb. (6 oz).
    Add your infused oil or dried herbs. Boil for about 20 minutes.

3. Strain any dried herbs from the oil using the cheesecloth, or another filter. Wipe off any herb detritus and add the clear oil back into the pot. If you're only using infused oil, go directly onto the next step.

4. Put the pot of oil back onto medium heat.

5. 2 Tablespoons of honey. Stir in the honey until it is completely combined.

6. ¼ cup beeswax (2 oz), in pellets or cut into pieces. Add to the heated oil. Stir continuously, so all the wax is combined.

7. Pour into the sterile glass jars or another container.

8. If you are adding essential oils, add a few drops to each jar and stir it in well with a chopstick.

9. Allow the salve to cool, occasionally stirring in the jar, so it cools evenly.

10. Seal tightly once it is thoroughly cooled.

If you would prefer a thicker consistency for the final salve, add a little more beeswax to the mixture while it is on medium heat.

Basic Cream Recipe

This cream should keep for up to a month or a little longer if refrigerated.

1. In a double-boiler set to medium heat, combine ¾ cup (12 oz) carrier oil (olive, coconut, jojoba, or infused oil) and ½-1 oz (2 tablespoons) beeswax. Stir continuously until the beeswax is melted.

2. Pour the oil blend into a blender and let cool. At room temperature, it turns cloudy and is ready for the next step.

3. Turn the blender onto high.

4. Slowly stream 1 cup (8 oz) of distilled water or rosewater into the center of the blender's mix to emulsify the ingredients. Don't let your blender overheat as it will remelt the wax and stop the emulsification process. Allow your blender to cool down before continuing if it overheats.

5. Stop adding water when the mix turns white and stiff.

6. Add in essential oil—just 2 to 5 drops depending on the strength; 2 drops for strong oils and 5 drops for milder oils such as lavender and rose. Don't add too much essential oil if you're using an infused oil.

7. Pour the cream into clean, sterile jars or containers.

8. Seal thoroughly.

Basic Methods for Infusing Oil

There are four ways to infuse oil. Two require heat, and two don't. You'll know your oil is infused when it takes on the color and scent of the herb or spice. Most infused oils should be fine to use for two months up to a year. When the oil goes rancid (the smell and consistency will change) or it develops mold, it's time to discard it.

Cold Method One—4 to 6 Weeks

1. Fill a jar (mason jars are best) or bottle with a herb of your choice till it is about ⅔ full.

2. Fill the bottle to the top with olive oil or another carrier such as coconut oil. Ensure all the herbs are covered.

3. Store in a cool, dark place for the next 4 to 6 weeks.

4. Shake the bottle often.

5. When the oil is done, strain the herbs out using cheesecloth or a coffee filter.

6. Decant into sterile glass bottles, label and store in a cool place or refrigerate.

Cold Method Two—Just over 24 hours

1. Smash or grind 1 oz (28g) of dried herbs into a rough powder. Place in a jar or bottle.

2. Pour a ½ oz (15 ml) of whole grain alcohol such as vodka into the bottle.

3. Shake the jar or mix the herbs and alcohol until the herbs look like damp soil.

4. Leave to steep for 24 hours.

5. Place herbs in a blender. Add at least 8 oz (1 cup) of carrier oil of your choice. Add more oil to cover the herbs if necessary.

6. Blend for about 5 minutes.

7. Strain the oil into a glass container, then decant for storage. Label the oil and expected expiration date.

Warm Method One—2 to 4 weeks

This method uses the same process as Cold Method One, but instead of leaving it in the pantry or other cool, dark place, we place it in the sun. Stand the infusing jar or bottle on a sunny windowsill or another sunny spot. Shake the bottle every now and then. The oil should be infused in two to four weeks. The longer you leave it on the windowsill, the stronger your infusion will be.

NB! Take care with the carrier oil you use for this method. Olive oil and coconut oil work best, while other oils such as grapeseed or rosehip oil may spoil. Covering the bottle with a paper bag or using smoked bottles may get you the best results.

Warm Method Two—Between 30 minutes and three days

This method requires a stove or crockpot.

1. Place 8 oz (1 cup) carrier oil and 6 oz (¼ cup) dried herbs in a saucepan, a double boiler, or a crockpot. Ensure the herbs are fully covered and that they are about 2 inches (5 cm) over the herbs.

2. Either place the herbs over a low heat 100 F (37 C) for 1 to 5 hours or on medium heat for about 20 minutes, ensuring the herbs aren't frying. If you have the time, you can leave the infusing oil on a constant heat of low in a crockpot for 48 to 72 hours to get a more potent infusion.

3. Allow the oil to cool, then strain using a filter or cheesecloth.

4. Decant into sterile glass bottles or jars and label with contents, date produced and expected expiration date.

Tinctures and Tonics

Tinctures and tonics are much the same as infusions, except that a tincture is always made with an alcohol or glycerin base.

They are usually administered by a dropper as it's important to only ingest small amounts of tinctures. **The usual safe daily dosage is usually 2,5ml or ½ a teaspoon twice a** *day.* *Tinctures can be diluted in water, in tea, in fruit juice, or even in sparkling water.*

Store tinctures in small tinted bottles to keep them longer.

Basic Tincture Method Using Alcohol

Alcohol-based tinctures can keep up to four to five years if stored well in a cool, dry place out of sunlight.

1. Fill a mason jar with dried herbs—not too coarse—until the jar is about ½ full.

2. Add the alcohol until the jar is full and all the herbs are entirely covered.

3. Ensure there is not too much air between the lid and the alcohol.

4. Cover the top of the jar with a paper sandwich bag or parchment paper.

5. Close the jar with a metal lid, so it is airtight.

6. Gently shake the bottle so the herbs can float in the liquid.

7. Store the jar in a pantry or other cool, dark area.

8. Shake the jar a few times each day.

9. Check that the herbs are always completely covered by alcohol as they may evaporate. If the alcohol level drops, top it up with as much alcohol as required.

10. Your tincture should be ready in about 6-8 weeks.

11. Strain the herbs with cheesecloth or a mesh strainer and funnel them into a tinted bottle.

12. Label the tincture carefully and use sparingly. Include a list of herbs used and the alcohol details on each label. Also include directions for use.

Note: If you are using fresh herbs, fill the jar to about ⅔ full, then add alcohol to fill the rest of the jar. Ensure fresh herbs are finely chopped.

Tincture Method Using Glycerin or Apple Cider Vinegar

If you would like an alcohol-free tincture, glycerin provides a sweeter and more palatable alternative but will spoil faster. ***Glycerin-based tinctures will keep for just over a year.***

Another alcohol-free option is to use the recipe above and substitute the alcohol with apple cider vinegar.

1. Mix ¾ cup vegetable glycerin with ¼ cup distilled or boiled water. Set aside.

2. Half fill a jar with dried herbs. If you're using fresh herbs, chop finely and fill the jar about ⅔ full.

3. Add the glycerin mixture into the jar, ensuring the jar is filled and the herbs are fully covered.

4. Store the bottle in a cool, dry place such as a pantry.

5. Shake the bottle every day.

6. After 4-6 weeks, your tincture is ready.

7. Strain all plant material out using a mesh strainer or coffee filter.

8. Funnel the tincture into tinted bottles.

9. Label with all the details: date bottled, ingredients, glycerin to water ratio, dosage instructions, and expected expiry date.

To make a tonic, dilute a tincture in distilled water, or add 2.5ml to a glass of juice, or tea of your choice.

Bruises and Scrapes Salve

For use on scrapes, minor cuts, and minor burns, diaper rash, and eczema.

You will need basic ingredients of the Basic Salve recipe, with these substitutes for the herbs and essential oil.

- 6 oz (¼ cup) comfrey, dried

- 6 oz (¼ cup) calendula, dried

- 6 oz (¼ cup) oregon grape root (optional)

- 5 to 10 drops lavender essential oil

To make it: Use the basic salve recipe and use a ¼ cup of dried herbs to every ½ cup or carrier oil.

Sunscreen

Any natural sunscreen needs to contain either zinc oxide or titanium dioxide to effectively block the sun's rays. Otherwise, you will have a sun filter cream instead of a sunblock cream. It is also hard to determine the efficiency of DIY Sunscreen as the UVB/UVA filtering will differ greatly depending on ingredients used and blends. Therefore, SPF factors will be variable. Also, homemade sunscreens are not waterproof. Therefore, further steps to prevent and minimize sunburn must be taken. The best sun protection remains covering up.

You will need:

- 1 cup shea butter

- ¼ cup jojoba oil or sweet almond oil (carrier oil)

- ¼ cup pure aloe vera (minimum 50% aloe vera)

- 2 to 3 tablespoons zinc oxide, powdered

- 25 drops of walnut extract oil

To make it:

1. In a double-boiler or saucepan, heat the shea butter, carrier oil, and walnut extract oil over medium heat.

2. Remove from heat when all the shea butter is melted and all the oils are well combined.

3. Allow the oil mixture to cool.

4. When cool, stir in aloe vera.

5. When the mixture is thoroughly cooled, stir in zinc oxide until it's all well combined.

6. Decant into jars or sterile containers for use.

Note: To have a thicker sunscreen cream, add in some beeswax. To make a spray instead of a cream, leave out the shea butter, adding more carrier oil, and once the oils have cooled, add more aloe vera until you can spray from a bottle easily.

Witch Hazel Wipes

Witch Hazel is a great antiseptic, antibacterial, antifungal, astringent, antimicrobial, and anti-inflammatory. Using wipes to help clean scrapes, cuts, bruises, and around open wounds is a swift and easy solution. These can also be used to treat sunburn, hemorrhoids, stings, and insect bites, and minor rashes.

These wipes might dry out after a few weeks, so it's best to use them quickly.

You will need:

- witch hazel (store-bought or infuse your own)

- essential oil of your choice. Lavender, peppermint, lemongrass, basil, rosemary or sage work well.

- aloe vera gel (optional)

- cotton cosmetic pads or cotton rounds

- airtight storage jar or container, or resealable airtight plastic bag.

To make it: Mix the 4 to 6 drops of essential oil into about 2 oz (¼ cup) with hazel. Add 1 oz (30ml) of aloe vera to the solution if you are using it. Place the cotton swabs and wipes in the airtight container. Gently pour the solution over the wipes. Ensure the swabs are wet through, but not to the point of dripping. Seal the container.

Note: You can also infuse witch hazel much as you infuse oil by using Cold Method One. However, the infusion is best refrigerated and may not be suitable for long-term storage in a first aid kit. It would be best used to treat rashes and other short-term irritations topically for a few days.

Anti-Itch Salve

You will need basic ingredients of the Basic Salve recipe, with these substitutes for the herbs and essential oil.

- plantain infused oil (make your own or store-bought)

- essential oils. Lavender, lemongrass, tea tree oil, and peppermint work well.

To make it: Follow the **Basic Salve Recipe**, skipping the addition of herbs and the straining of the oil. Once the infused oil is heated, skip straight to adding in the beeswax.

Note: The addition of peppermint, lemongrass, basil, or lavender, may also work as an insect repellent for certain insects such as centipedes and wasps.

Burn Salve

You will need: basic ingredients of the **Basic Salve** recipe with these substitutes and additions. It's best to use coconut oil for this recipe.

- Additional raw honey

- aloe vera

- lavender essential oil (optional)

To make it: Heat ½ cup (4 oz) coconut oil on medium heat. Stir in ¾ cup (6 oz) of honey. Add 1 to 2 oz of beeswax to get to the consistency you desire. Stir until the beeswax has melted. Pour oil into a dish to cool. When the oil is cool, stir in 2 to 4 oz of aloe vera. Add essential oil. Stir slowly and thoroughly. Decant into storage jars or containers and label.

Rash Cream

You will need: basic ingredients of the **Basic Cream** recipe, with these substitutes for the herbs and essential oil.

- ⅓ cup aloe vera

- ¾ cup infused oil of marshmallow root, chamomile, and lemon balm. Optional herbs or substitute herbs could be calendula or lavender.

- 1 to 2 drops of essential oil. Tea tree oil, lavender, or peppermint work well

- ⅔ cup distilled water

To make it: Heat the infused oil and the beeswax and stir until the beeswax has melted. Remove from heat. When the oil is at room temperature, combine the water and aloe vera. Slowly blend the water into the oil using a blender as in the Basic Cream recipe. Once the emulsification is done, add in the essential oil. Decant into jars or containers and label the cream.

Peppermint Tincture

Peppermint is great for treating abdominal pains, indigestion and helping relieve headaches. It is also antibacterial. However, care must be taken if a person is on medication as it does interact with a range of medications. While peppermint can also be applied topically to help relieve congestion (as you do with a salve), children and infants should not be administered peppermint at all.

To make peppermint tincture, follow the basic tincture recipe of your choice.

Disinfectant and Hand Sanitizers

If you run out of disinfectants or hand sanitizers, you can also make your own. However, they may not be as effective as approved store-bought products, but they are useful in a bind. These recipes are particularly helpful if you are in a remote location or your area is under an extended general quarantine.

Some of the ingredients in these recipes may damage or stain unsealed surfaces such as granite or wood. However, they are good for disinfecting daily items if no bleach is available.

NB! These recipes contain alcohol and are highly flammable! Store safely away from heat sources. Store them in child-safe places.

Disinfectant Spray

You will need:

- ½ cup white distilled vinegar

- 1 ½ cup alcohol (highest proof Vodka available or rubbing alcohol that is a minimum of 70% proof)

- 50 drops lavender or tea tree essential oil

To make it: Combine the essential oil and alcohol in a large enough spray bottle. Shake the bottle to mix the two thoroughly. It is best to use a figure-eight motion. Then add the vinegar and mix thoroughly again. The disinfectant is now ready for use.

Two Step Bleach-free Disinfecting

You will need:

- hydrogen peroxide

- white distilled vinegar

- a spray bottle

- a spray cap to fit the hydrogen peroxide bottle if possible

Warning! Never mix hydrogen peroxide and vinegar together in a bottle! The fumes released when they are combined are poisonous and can damage your health.

How to do it: First use the hydrogen peroxide on a surface by spraying it. Let it lie for about 5 minutes. Wipe off the area thoroughly. Next, spray on the vinegar. Let it lie for about another 5 minutes. Then wipe off the vinegar. The surface is now disinfected of the most common illness-causing organisms.

Hand Sanitizer Method One

Remember to wash your hands first, as the disinfectant cannot do its job through dirt, grease and other oils. If no water is available, wipe your hands down first with antibacterial wipes such as the witch hazel wipes.

Ensure the alcohol you're using isn't diluted so that the 60-70% alcohol concentration is maintained in the end product.

When mixing hand sanitizers, ensure the surface you're working on is disinfected, as well as your hands and all the equipment you're using.

Don't touch the hand sanitizer liquid when decanting it into bottles. Allow the bottles to sit for 72 hours if possible.

You will need:

- ½ cup aloe vera gel

- 1 cup ethanol or isopropyl alcohol (rubbing alcohol 99% proof)

- 10-20 drops of essential oil. Peppermint, cloves, lavender, or tea tree oil work well. Lemon juice can be substituted for essential oils.

To make it: Mix the essential oil into the aloe vera gel in a large plastic bottle or a bucket. Add the alcohol. Mix thoroughly or, if it's in a bottle, shake the bottle gently. Decant the sanitizer into a bottle with a screw cap or a hand dispenser. If you'd like to use this recipe for a spray, add a little more undiluted alcohol until you get a spraying consistency.

Note: To make this sanitizer in larger or smaller quantities, simply stick to the 1 part aloe vera to 2 parts 99% proof alcohol.

Hand Sanitizer Method Two

You will need:

- ½ cup alcohol highest proof vodka (100% or over) or rubbing alcohol (99%)

- 1 tsp vegetable glycerin (also called glycerine or glycerol)

- 10-20 drops of essential oils. Lavender, spruce, lemon, citrus, eucalyptus, or chamomile all work well.

To make it: Mix the glycerin and essential oils well together in a 4 oz bottle. Add the alcohol until the bottle is full. Cap the bottle and shake gently to mix.

Alternatives to the First Aid Kit Material

Burns

- If you don't have water to cool the burn, use any other cool liquid such as juice, beer, milk, etc. Any harmless liquid will do as your priority is to cool the area until you have access to cold, running water.

- Remember, the burn should be cooled for at least twenty minutes for the treatment to be effective.

- If you don't have cling film to cover the burn, use a clean plastic bag such as a carrier bag, freezer bag, sandwich bag, or similar. These items won't stick to the burn and will prevent infection.

- Plastic bags are well suited to covering a burned hand or foot.

Broken Bones

If you don't know what padding to use for broken bones, use clothing, blankets, etc. Or hold the injured part yourself. A half-rolled magazine held by duct tape can serve as a makeshift cast or protection for a limb for short-term transport. Popsicle sticks make good finger splints.

Heavy Bleeding

If you don't have dressing pads to put on the wound, use a clean t-shirt, or clean tea towel, sanitary pads, or clamp the person's hand over their injury.

Your priority is to put pressure on the wound to stop or slow down the bleeding.

Diabetic Emergency

If you don't have glucose tablets, use orange juice, a few sugar cubes, candy, or packets of sugar. Alternatively, use any regular fizzy drink, except diet beverages.

Head Injury

If you don't have any ice cubes, use a packet of frozen peas wrapped in a tea towel. Alternatively, use clothing soaked in cold water and wrung out. A half-collapsed baseball cap can be used as a temporary neck brace. Push the back of the cap in so the front of the cap with the peak creates a cradle (just as many stores stack them). Fit the cap with the peak facing the person's chest so that the rest of the cap cradles their chin. Secure the cap with duct tape.

Eye Injury

Use a paper cup to protect the eye if no eye shield is available. Secure it with duct tape. Ensure you don't tape over hair, if possible.

Hypothermia

If there are no blankets or space blankets available, consider using aluminum foil if it is at hand.

CONCLUSION

Well done! You're now equipped to face and help a distressed person through a variety of emergencies.

You have your list of items and medication you can either buy and sometimes make yourself for your first aid kits and responses. In fact, you have more than one method to handle skin infections and promote healing. You can even improvise aids like a sling or a splint when needed.

You have your steps to follow in both minor and major emergencies, whether an insect bite, a minor burn, or a major burn or hypothermia. You even know how to identify and treat emergencies related to chronic illnesses, such as a person experiencing a heart attack or suffering from hypoglycemia.

Most importantly, you know to keep calm, how to keep yourself safe while assisting someone, and how to manage the situation until professional help arrives.

Your next step is to get certified in first aid techniques such as CPR or expanding your knowledge in preparing natural remedies that are safe and effective for home and first-aid use.

We like to keep a batch of multi-purpose herbal salves such as the Bruises and Cuts Salve on hand for everyday use. We also encourage you to experiment with these homemade preparations, so you have one that is uniquely suited to your and your family's needs.

As a parting note, we'd like you to keep some things in mind.

Remember

Communicate with the person you're treating from the moment you approach them. This will reassure both of you. Explain what you intend to do—the treatment—and tell them what you're doing at each step unless you're doing CPR. Keep your voice low and steady, and if they are agitated, this will also help them calm down and follow any instructions you may need to give them.

Use gentleness to attend to younger children and babies. Treat them as fragile and try not to let your sense of urgency result in your use of forceful movements when dealing with them. Children may need more reassurance and patience if they are conscious. It will be worth taking a moment to talk to them and explain that you mean no harm, and only want to help them. If their parent or an older sibling is present, let them talk to the child. Keep your voice calm and friendly while working with the child and don't let them sense any worry you might feel about their condition.

Only use medication from a first aid kit that has not expired and herbal remedies that still smell good.

Self-care

Self-care is vitally important before, during, and after you've given first aid in an emergency. After all, if you are ill or experiencing extreme anxiety throughout, you cannot be as effective as you'd like to be or help as you might wish.

Before you begin attending to a person in distress, do all you can to ensure your safety as well as theirs. For instance, if you have a bright jacket or flashlight, it's a good idea to use it or turn it on if you are attending to someone in dim light at the side of the road. Or if you're helping someone in freezing weather, you can also take a minute to wear your down coats and pull on a hat or beanie and wear gloves, so you don't get frostbite or worse. Also, be aware of your physical limitations and your own needs. Don't be afraid to ask for help from bystanders or others present. For example, if you are petite and a giant of a person is choking, don't attempt the Heimlich maneuver. Thump their back between the shoulder blades instead or call the attention of someone bigger in stature to assist.

While you're attending the person, no-one expects you to be super-human. Do the best you can, but if you're exhausted and can't continue chest compressions, it's okay to take a break and let someone else take over, or if you're alone, to try reviving the person again if you feel that's possible. When you've done your best, there's nothing else anyone can ask of you.

If you fear contamination or have a cold, it's okay to ask a conscious person in distress to help dress their wound. Always wear gloves and other protective gear if you have them available. Use a pocket mask or face mask where possible if you're giving CPR.

If you feel you can't do a technique, look for help or a safe alternative. Remember, your priority is to preserve life, prevent deterioration, and promote recovery. Your priority isn't about getting top marks in a book exam.

During and after your care of the person, practicing breathing or relaxation techniques will help you stay calm and keep you alert and focused.

After the incident, you may run through a range of emotional responses to your experience and even that of the person, particularly if you are very empathetic. This is normal. If the feelings of wellbeing, confidence, and gratitude continue, know that you've earned them and enjoy them. However, if you feel anxiety, are hyper alert, experience nightmares, stress, other negative emotions, or take on the experience of the person that you've helped, you need to talk to someone to fully process the experience and find your balance again.

Discuss your experience with a good friend, your doctor or other professional. If you are in contact with someone else who was at the scene, you can help each other process through your feelings and responses. If you have no-one to talk to, journal your experiences and your responses.

For the next few days or weeks after the incident, ensure you get enough sleep, avoid alcohol and caffeine, and eat healthy. Exercise will help you find your balance as well.

A FINAL NOTE

We'd like to take this opportunity to acknowledge your bravery and resilience. Stepping up to assist a distressed person takes courage as well as knowledge. Your quick actions can not only help the distressed person or save their life, but your care and observation also assist the medical professionals who will eventually arrive to take over the situation, and for this, we thank you.

We also thank you for making the world a better place for us all. While we at Small Footprint Press do our best to help everyone prepare for emergencies and prevent as many as possible from happening, we like knowing there are people out there, like you, willing to lend a helping hand when needed.

Go well and be safe!

***

If you've found this book helpful, please leave a review on Amazon.

THE WORST-CASE SURVIVAL BOOK FOR DISASTER PREPAREDNESS

"Extinction is the rule. Survival is the exception."

- Carl Sagan

Introduction

You will, no doubt, have many reasons for becoming a prepper. In recent years, we have seen the effects of climate change in our backyards, from floods to fires to rising food prices. At the same time, we are watching as the fat cats at the top steal and pillage, leaving little for those at the bottom.

It is just a matter of time before solar flares, financial disasters, storms, hurricanes, earthquakes, and pandemics become a normal way of living for us. Unfortunately, many non-preppers may want to go on believing that things will turn out okay after all, but rising sea levels, melting glaciers, hotter temperatures, and new viruses tell a different story.

The truth of the matter is that, in this new world about to descend on us, the 'haves' and the 'have nots' will be even more clearly divided. Unlike the world we have now, in the new world, the 'haves' will be preppers: those who had the good sense to prepare for a disaster before it finally came.

We are all holding on to human civilization by a thread. You will have noticed people still buying their flat-screen TVs and heavily processed foods, ignoring the evidence right before their eyes. But you know the truth, that both you and your family are in danger.

It may not seem like it to people who are too busy entertaining their lives away, but, as an astute prepper, you know that hundreds of potentially life-threatening situations can change life as we know it–even in an instant. Those in the know realize that prepping is the only way to be truly prepared for anything: it is the only way that gives us the best chance of survival.

Let's face it, you have no excuse not to prepare for disaster. This is the easiest time in history to be a prepper, thanks to technological advances and recent developments in the prepping community, developments that we will share with you in subsequent chapters. As a prepper, you have no excuse not to take control over disaster by preparing well for yourself and your family.

To support you on your journey and give you that much-needed sense of control over your environment, we have written this detailed and essential preparation guidebook to give you back control. Not only will you gain back control over your survival with this comprehensive guide, but you will also ward off terror and fear of the unknown. You will find that once you understand how to prepare for disaster, the fear of doom will no longer control you.

In essence, this book aims to free you from fear by teaching you practical skills for survival. So, how will we achieve this? Simple. We know you are a survivor. What we want to do is help you on your way to unlocking your natural capabilities by educating you on the steps you need to take to achieve this. These are easy-to-remember steps presented through the P.O.S.S.E.S.S framework.

- **P**racticing self-reliance always.

- **O**btaining traditional cooking and medical skills.

- **S**toring food and water securely and safely.

- **S**ynthesizing an off-grid waste system.

- **E**quipping yourself for self-defense against threats.

- **S**urviving when shit hits the fan.

- **S**urviving disaster and collapse.

This framework empowers you to check how many essential survival skills you have picked up for when disaster comes or shit really hits the fan! Indeed, as you go through this book, you will find that each chapter presents you with a similar framework to help you easily find the answers you are seeking. Each framework is there to bring you a memorable answer to all your prepper problems.

By reading this book, you will first learn how to start your journey of living off-grid and how to prepare for a variety of catastrophes or events which would require self-sufficiency. You will also learn other essential skills that you need to survive in a disaster. Each chapter represents a distinct element of prepping that you will need to consider to be well-prepared, as well as tips on implementing this effectively.

Not just content with bringing you tips and guides, we will also aim to give you "practices" for disasters. We will illustrate to you prepping scenarios for a variety of disasters, including information on how prepping in advance may save your life in those situations. We will also bring you practical guidance on how to ensure that you have constant water and food supplies in whatever disaster scenario you find yourself in.

Don't fret! We know you want to protect yourself and your family, so we are here to teach you how by bringing you the basics of self-defense strategies and essential weaponry. Expect to learn the pros and cons of different types of shelter, for the wilderness and for home, as well as the how-to for making a 72-hour kit bag with all the essentials that you need.

By the end of this book, you will be able to create your own emergency plan, including different roles for yourself and your family. In addition, you will be introduced to the concept of homesteading, with tips on how you can start to implement this in your own home.

Also, all the guidance and tips in this book are specifically tailored so that they can be used anywhere in the world. We aim to reach as many preppers as possible, so we have also ensured that our tips and guidance can be followed by all preppers, regardless of income level.

You will not find us recommending unnecessary high-tech or expensive survival equipment. Rather, we believe the core value of the survival prepper is to keep it as simple as possible, using as many everyday items as possible to improve your chances of survival.

We recognize that you may have done some previous research of your own on disaster prepping, so we are not here to bring you the standard disaster prepping advice. Instead, we have come prepared with new, inexpensive solutions to many of your disaster prep problems–solutions that you will find nowhere else. You can expect to gain insightful knowledge of unusual prepping techniques, many of which may be new and exciting to you.

You are not alone. Whatever your reason for prepping, you can be assured that you have picked up the perfect book that will keep you one step ahead of disaster. By the end of this book, you will feel more confident in your preparations for any disaster that may befall your part of the world and will be able to cope with a variety of situations that would catch out even experienced preppers.

Many more people are seeing the light these days and realizing the extreme benefits of being a prepper. Indeed, even celebrities, with all their wealth and connections, are coming to their senses and becoming preppers. Celebrities like Ryan Seacrest, Jamie Lee Curtis, Roseanne Barr, Zooey Deschanel, and Nathan Fillion are all self-proclaimed preppers who have all seen the need. They know that their wealth and connections will not be enough to survive. After all, disaster is the great equalizer!

When push comes to shove and we all have to survive, it is every man and woman for themselves. So, if you're ready to begin your prepping journey and to become more self-reliant, more self-assured, more confident, and less anxious, then let's begin! You are the fittest and you will survive, beginning with learning the different disaster scenarios which every prepper may face.

Who is Small Footprint Press?

Small Footprint Press, established amidst the pandemic, is a self-publishing company of experts that aims to promote sustainable survival–equipping you to live a sustainable, conscious, and independent lifestyle to make the world a better place for yourself and future generations to come.

As the world progresses, we believe that the importance of sustainable survival becomes more and more evident. Our planet faces various challenges, including climate change, dwindling resources, population growth, and pandemics. To secure a bright future for our children *now* is the time we must take steps to save our planet.

We accomplish this by simply empowering you to prepare for potential disasters for yourself and your loved ones. Gone are the days when you stress about the day of the unknown!

Our books are a collaboration of different authors, each with their perspective and expertise. This makes for a well-rounded book that covers various topics in depth, ensuring the highest quality standards. It also makes for a more engaging read, as each author brings their unique style to the table.

Similarly, orchestras comprise different instruments, each with its unique sound and purpose. Once these instruments play as one in harmony, the result is extraordinary.

We believe that one way to bridge a community of people with a shared purpose and values is through books! In this community, you will build genuine relationships, share similar experiences, and be empowered to take action.

You are not alone. There's something special about a journey taken with others. Whether exploring a new city or embarking on a long hike, sharing the experience with others makes you enjoy the journey more than the destination.

So allow us to join you in your journey to a compelling life of sustainable survival! Interested in joining our cause? Download your FREE resources at the beginning of the book!

Chapter One:
Prepping 101

If you are new to disaster preparation, you may ask yourself what it is all about. Sure, you have a general idea of what it entails, but what exactly does being a "prepper" mean? Does it mean preparing for the end of the world, pandemics, war, or natural disasters?

There are so many forms of disaster that, for a beginner, it may be difficult to pinpoint what exactly this community is about. Believe it or not, some people even prep for a zombie apocalypse! So how do we narrow down what we mean when we say "prepper"? Well, using the framework P.R.E.P.P.E.R, you can easily understand that prepping empowers you to:

- **P**rotect yourself and your loved ones.

- **R**isk-assess your chance of survival when disaster strikes.

- **E**vade deep pain and suffering caused by a disaster.

- **P**osition yourself as a leader in the community.

- **P**repare yourself mentally for survival.

- **E**ncourage your natural human instinct for survival.

- **R**espond to threats with appropriate force.

As you read through this chapter, you will find ways in which being a P.R.E.P.P.E.R helps you find common life-saving solutions against disaster and its accompanying problems. The one thing you can tell from the framework is that a prepper does not hide from the harsh truths and cold realities of the world. A prepper knows that civilizations, societies, and communities can, and have, collapsed in the past—whether temporarily or permanently.

Rather than leave it up to chance and false hope that they will never face a collapse in their lifetime, a prepper stands tall to take control of their life. A prepper values their survival, and hence, does the hard work necessary to survive. A prepper knows that the civilizations we humans build for ourselves are precarious at best. One flood, one night of riots, or one pandemic is all it takes to wipe it all away for an extended period.

Being a prepper is simply common sense. You are honoring and following your natural human instinct for survival, an instinct that has been developed and fine-tuned over many generations.

So, whether you prepare for water scarcity, food scarcity, financial difficulties, self-defense, a pandemic, security, loss of power, or even a zombie apocalypse, what matters is that you are following your natural human instinct for survival because you never know when the system will fail you and you will need a back-up plan.

We can say, then, that a prepper is a responsible, enterprising risk-assessor who creates their own survival insurance against a rainy day. One of the easiest ways to become a prepper is to follow a preparedness pyramid. A preparedness pyramid is a pyramid that shows you all the different emergencies you can prepare for. It works like any other pyramid.

On the bottom are the most basic/common events to prepare for based on the likelihood of them happening. Nearing the top are those events that are less likely to occur but will need more extensive preparation if you are to survive.

A preparedness pyramid is typically structured into these five levels, with level 1 at the base and level 5 at the peak:

1. Basic prepping

Basic prepping is prepping for basic emergencies that will be typically resolved after a few hours or days at most. For example, having emergency flashlights at home in case of a sudden power outage. Basic prepping is also for everyday emergencies that you are so used to that you may not even consider them being emergencies, such as ensuring you have some cash on you at all times in case you cannot use your debit/credit card.

2. Temporary setbacks

Temporary setbacks typically set us back a few weeks or months before we can bounce back. Your roof may need extensive repairs, or you may need to be off work for a couple of weeks. Temporary setbacks typically have a low financial impact and can be solved with an emergency fund.

3. Weather, recession and injuries

Weather, recession, and injuries can be classified as more serious setbacks. They can set you back months and even years. A freak storm could cause you to lose your home, for example, or you may need to be admitted into hospital for a few months, unable to work. The best prep method for these disasters is, of course, insurance.

4. Disaster and collapse

What happens if society collapses? What happens if you experience a major financial/geopolitical crisis or a natural disaster? Your primary worry would be how you would survive the first night and subsequent nights after.

Imagine you hear that enemy troops are marching into your city. You need to head for the nearest border. You will save plenty of time if you already have your survival kit packed for the future, including supplies to last you during the treacherous journey.

When preparing for disaster and collapse, you need to ensure you can survive a week without regular amenities, such as working supermarkets selling food and readily available running water. Let us give you a scenario: if the national grid is damaged thanks to a flood, then you will still have electricity until the issue is fixed thanks to your prior preparation!

Let's look at another scenario: perhaps you need to evacuate to a safer area after an earthquake but are trapped thanks to rubble. You have enough supplies to last a couple of weeks. However, you will need other things apart from food and drink if you are to meet your needs. If you are trapped in a disaster zone, one of the greatest tools for survival that you will have at your disposal is information. But what happens if you have no means of communicating with the outside world because the electricity is down? In this case, a power bank will help you charge your phone and any other devices that you can use to communicate with the outside world. Indeed, your power bank could end up saving your life if you have enough power in your mobile phone to reach emergency/rescue services.

As the disastrous effects of climate change become a regular occurrence and geopolitical tensions rise all over the world, a level four preparation is a matter of life and death.

Conversely, while disaster preparation requires short-term planning, surviving a financial or political collapse requires long-term planning. After society collapses, you can no longer rely on the government and on businesses to provide you with stability. By preparing, you offer yourself stability in an unstable world.

For example, an emergency fund (a stash of physical cash) could help you to purchase food during an economic depression, especially if bank cards stop working. The fact is that collapse brings with it less reliable power, an unstable supply of drinking water, and very little food. Hence, the more self-sufficient you are, the more likely you are to survive. In the case of collapse, self-sufficiency includes things like growing your own food, having an emergency food stash, and having a way to filter water and make it safe for drinking (as discussed further in other chapters).

5. SHTF (Shit Hits The Fan)

Level five, or "shit hits the fan" helps you prepare for the worst that could possibly happen. This could be things like a deadly pandemic, a nuclear disaster, or a deep societal collapse where civilization has completely broken down. This is usually the case when war breaks out or international conflict escalates, resulting in war crimes, something we have seen happen more and more in recent decades. In this scenario, there is no law, and it is truly survival of the fittest.

Have you seen those disaster movies where one man or woman is trying to survive in a post-collapse or post-apocalyptic world? You will notice that the protagonist is always well-prepared while characters who aren't well-prepared usually die at the beginning of the movie. The same happens in real life. Those who survived war zones in Europe during the 20th century often had one of two things on their side: (1) being prepared and (2) luck.

Another important reason for being well-prepared is that when the shit hits the fan, go back to the most primitive survival methods humans have. Unfortunately, we rely on technology too much nowadays. The problem with our reliance on technology is that technology requires a lot of processes to keep it working.

Even the simplest part not working can cause everything to shut down. So, a wealthy oligarch might think they are fine in their fortress, complete with a cinema, two double-door fridges, and the highest speed internet. But if the electric generator stops working, and they don't know how to fix it or are not prepared with the tools needed to fix it, the shit really will hit the fan.

A good prepper prepares for all eventualities and is certain of survival, even when technology fails. During a disaster, the everyday tools we take for granted become as precious as gold. You may have a gun for shooting prey for food, however, you won't want to waste a finite number of bullets on killing a rabbit for dinner. As a result, a simple rope and knife will become your most prized possessions since they help you trap and kill animals for food.

As a prepper, it is important to begin with the base of the pyramid because preparing for the basics gives you a chance of surviving any doomsday scenario. For example, packing basic survival gear like batteries, water, and a first aid kit will keep you alive longer than not doing so, no matter the situation you are in.

Levels 1-3 are regarded as "common sense" preparation among preppers. It is common sense to have insurance in case of emergencies. It is also common sense to have emergency funds to cover temporary setbacks in life. This book will focus on level 4 (disaster/collapse) and level 5 (SHTF) because these emergencies require more than "common sense." They require more expert skills and knowledge reserved only for those intelligent enough to seek it.

WHAT AM I PREPPING FOR?

Reading the beginning of this chapter, you can already tell that there are different disaster scenarios that you may face at any moment. Likewise, you know by now that there are wonderful benefits of prepping for survival and becoming self-reliant. But before you can determine what to prep, you must first understand what you are prepping for. To determine the cure, you must first diagnose the illness to know what challenges you are facing. So, what are you prepping for?

There are six major disasters that preppers typically prepare for. They are:

1. Natural disasters

The first thing that comes to mind when prepping for disaster is probably natural disasters. Natural disasters are a big part of the human experience, occurring with alarming frequency. As climate change worsens, we have seen bigger and more frequent natural disasters. From floods, to earthquakes, to hurricanes, to forest fires, natural disasters can destroy entire countries. They can also disrupt your power supply, communication, and food and water supply for a long time. Undeniably, they are a serious issue.

2. Artificial disasters

Artificial disasters are a much sadder experience than natural disasters because they are most often needlessly and accidentally caused. It is always best to treat artificial disasters as seriously as natural disasters because of their ability to destroy almost everything immediately.

Sometimes, artificial disasters can be more dangerous than natural disasters. One of the most destructive disasters that can befall any prepper is a nuclear power meltdown or a bomb explosion. These disasters are so dangerous, particularly because they have the power to cause deep pain and suffering, even for generations.

Think about how people say that it is better to die in a nuclear explosion than to live with the effects of radiation poisoning. The problem is, you don't get a say in that and you could have to face the consequences of surviving the initial blast.

Conversely, there are so many ways for a bomb explosion to hurt you, for example, glass shards exploding and hurling themselves into your body at full speed. There is hope, however, if you know how to protect yourself from the effects of artificial disasters, then you reduce your chances and intensity of pain and suffering.

What we can say definitely is that artificial disasters are just as dangerous as natural ones and should be taken just as seriously.

3. Social unrest

Social unrest is a constant threat to your survival. It usually manifests as protests, riots, walkouts, or wars. During times of social unrest, you cannot rely on society to work like clockwork, so your normal way of life becomes threatened. Take, for example, a nationwide truckers' strike. Truckers decide to walk out on a national scale for better conditions. As a result, food distribution becomes affected, leading to empty aisles at the supermarket.

If you are prepped with food to last you until the strike is over, you won't have to panic buy or become anxious when you cannot find any food at the supermarket. Let's take another example. If you and your family suddenly find yourselves near a bomb explosion and chaos erupts, you could easily become separated. There is safety in numbers, and separation also increases your chances of further disaster happening to one or more of you.

However, if you plan on what to do during emergencies, your training will kick in even during the chaos, and you can all stay safe together.

4. Biological warfare

Most countries today have nukes and biochemical weapons. We have seen, in recent years, that some national leaders are not scared of using these weapons against their own people and they wouldn't hesitate to use them as threats. If you want to survive, you must consider modern health hazards and prepare adequately for them.

5. Financial challenges

Saving has become a lost art today. Everyone wants to buy, buy, buy, but forget that there will come a time when they face financial difficulties. As a prepper, you are smart enough to resist the status quo, so you work hard to be free of debt in every way. You pour your money into canned food, gardening, green housing, and other ways to keep you alive when you meet future financial challenges. You are also savvy enough to recognize that it is much cheaper and much more self-reliant to produce your own food.

Sometimes, financial challenges come because of wider societal or financial problems that are not your fault. Rightfully, in these cases, you cannot control the value of your currency/currencies. However, a prepper knows that you must also stock up with things that can be used as barter if money becomes valueless.

6. Personal challenges

Life is filled with ups and downs. We all wish it was filled with just ups–in which case you wouldn't need to prep. A wise person sees the warning signs of trouble in the future and prepares for it. A foolish person blindly looks away and pretends it will not affect them. In fact, a foolish person will tell you that preparing for disaster is simply an overreaction.

However, even if you are lucky enough to avoid a major level 4 or 5 disaster, prepping is still a great idea because it allows you to survive the personal challenges with less stress and pain. Either way, the wise person wins!

Prepping for personal challenges is even more imperative if you have young children or other vulnerable people who depend on you. We hate to say it, but the truth is that we live in a 'dog eat dog world.' Nobody will come to rescue you or your family if you suffer personal challenges that set you back.

The fat cats in power often like to act as though they care just to get our votes. They often manipulate us into buying their products and creating more wealth for them by working in their factories. They make promises, but always disappoint us at the worst possible moment. Those in power will never come to your aid. Indeed, what will more than likely happen is that you will be blamed despite being a victim yourself.

As a prepper, you are too self-reliant to have your hand out to the government because you know they will fail you.

On the other hand, ordinary people will never turn against more powerful men and women. So, when you prep and shoulder personal challenges, you do not need to rely on anyone for help to get back up or survive. You show others you belong to a class of powerful people. Your strength immediately and naturally demands other people's respect, and as a result, your confidence soars.

Every single person on this Earth will face at least one of these events in their lifetime. It is safe to say we will probably all face more than one of these events in our lifetime. Since we live in a world where only the fittest survive, you are technically descended from the fittest. It is in your genes to survive!

In essence, we are the children of strong survivors and warriors. Therefore, it is nothing but an insult to take modern conveniences and technology for granted and waste your time sitting on the couch, eating a delivered pizza, and wasting electricity watching shows with no value on TV.

To honor those ancestors who suffered so you could be here today, it is your human duty to work hard to continue to use the survival skills that are now embedded in your DNA and to learn new skills that will enable your great-great-great-grandchild to survive too.

One of the greatest examples of not honoring your survival instinct happened during the COVID-19 pandemic. We all saw the footage of people fighting, scrambling, and rushing just to buy a 6-pack of toilet paper, a bottle of water, alcohol, and sanitizers. Before that, preppers were seen by the world as conspiracy nuts. But those of us who knew were not worried about that because we had a sense of dignity and personal pride.

Once people faced the almost apocalyptic nightmare of trying to survive during COVID, respect for our intelligence and our dignity grew. Here is what one journalist wrote during the height of the pandemic:

"You've heard of preppers, right? Survivalists? You know about their strange, apocalyptic beliefs: that a disaster could strike at any time, overwhelming first responders and the social safety net; that this crisis could disrupt supply chains, causing scarcity and panic and social breakdown; that authorities might invoke emergency powers and impose police curfews. Crazy theories like that.

"In fact, many perfectly reputable organizations—including the US federal government and the Red Cross—recommend Americans maintain extra food and emergency supplies. The Federal Emergency Management Agency (FEMA) advises keeping a two-week supply of food, as well as water, batteries, medical masks, first-aid supplies, and a battery-or hand-powered radio, among other things.

"In mainstream society, however, interest in prepping usually invites ridicule about bunkers and tin-foil hats. Preppers have spent years as the objects of our collective derision.

"Until now. Today, we're all preppers—or rather, wish we had been. Non-preppers have been caught in a rain shower without an umbrella. I don't know if preppers are laughing right now, but perhaps they're entitled to some vindication.

But I've come to respect the preppers' ethos of survival and preparedness. One of my friends is one, or at least on the spectrum. When coronavirus hit, he wasn't one of the millions of people scrambling for surgical masks; he already had them in his survival kit. He kept a few and gave the rest to elderly people" (Conroy, 2020).

If, by some chance, you still aren't convinced, here are some other compelling reasons for becoming a prepper:

1. You strengthen your community

Despite the COVID-19 pandemic, many people still aren't preppers today. After the buying and hoarding madness during the early months of the pandemic, most people were so desperate to return to normal that they forgot all about the usefulness of prepping, especially in case of another (inevitable) disaster.

As you saw in the article above, the prepper in that situation was able to take care of his community by providing surgical masks to the vulnerable in the community. When you are a prepper, you are a leader of your community because you are a chance for survival and a beacon of hope for those around you.

This may seem like an exaggeration, but think about it. If you have your own farm and can feed your neighbors' children during civil unrest, you become a beacon of hope for your neighbors until the unrest ends and they can go out and buy some more food. This leads us to the second reason why preppers are so useful to the world.

2. You foster peace and wellbeing

Think of the panic in your community if people cannot feed their children, the elderly, babies, pets, and any other vulnerable people? Think of how people may get desperate and resort to crime and violence. However, if you can provide rations, supplies, and tools, peace is restored in your community temporarily until authorities can restore a more stable peace and stability.

During the Blitz in London, Londoners often huddled in the underground to avoid German bomber planes. One particular time, a nursing mother was stuck with other mothers and children for weeks. Food was scarce and there would not be enough for even the children. The mothers decided to feed the nursing mother alone instead so that she could breastfeed all the babies and the children.

Because of their quick thinking and putting their supplies to good use, the crisis was averted. While it may not be wise (or legal) for every prepper in the world to keep a nursing mother in case of emergencies, raising animals is a great alternative for providing constant food, sustenance, and nutrition in times of crisis.

You also foster peace when you store goods—by not needing to panic buy in times of disaster. The more preppers in a society, the fewer people will be out and about panic buying. In turn, there will be more supplies to go around, thereby reducing the air of panic and fear among those who have not prepped and are desperate for supplies.

BENEFITS OF PREPPING

We have already inadvertently covered some of the benefits of prepping in this chapter, namely because they are so numerous. Likewise, here are some more surprising benefits of being a prepper:

1. Boosts your confidence

Being a prepper gives you a confidence boost and affects all other areas of your life. When you are a prepper, you essentially train yourself to be a leader; you teach yourself how to be responsible, even in moments of chaos. In the process, you also train yourself to be calm and to focus on what you and others need to do to survive.

This stoicism and responsibility naturally draw others to you, making you a leader. As a naturally elected leader, your self-confidence will rise and begin to affect other areas of your life, such as your work, your relationships, and your finances. Since people trust you for something as important as their survival, it makes you feel more capable and more trustworthy. Soon, you begin to act accordingly.

Confidence breeds success, which, in turn, reinforces your confidence. In any case, it is a win-win situation.

2. Your relationship with your family deepens

Thanks to your newfound confidence, your relationship with your family gets better. Doing drills together and prepping together also helps you spend time and bond. Finally, your family will feel happy and supported to know that you care enough about them to include them in your disaster preparation plans.

a. You feel less stressed and anxious on a day-to-day basis knowing that you and your family are prepared and protected.

b. You enjoy yourself.

The more you prep, the more you try new things that you may not have tried otherwise. You may want to try gardening or having your own greenhouse, to wean yourself from your reliance on supermarkets. You may also try animal husbandry (raising animals), fishing, camping, and hunting—earning you a new hobby sooner or later.

Prepping is a great way to stimulate your mind, stop boredom and even meet new people. There is always something else you can learn to improve your preparedness and survival skills, some of which will require you to meet with other people, such as learning how to fire a gun or learning how to hunt.

Even better, the more you socialize with strangers, the more likely your bartering and negotiation skills will also improve—skills you will need to survive a disaster. Think about how convincing someone to trust you enough to give you a lift during mass civil unrest could be the deciding factor in whether you survive or die.

3. You get fitter

You will need to be fit to survive in case of a disaster. You can't run from advancing enemy troops, for example, if you have not kept yourself in great shape before disaster strikes. Hence, prepping keeps you healthy, especially if you switch to growing and/or rearing your own organic produce.

a. You get the satisfaction of one day being the hero who saves others with your exceptional leadership skills.

b. Financial rewards.

You can make money on the side by selling produce from your gardens or your farm animals. You can also sell any surplus supplies you don't need (once you take care of your family and the vulnerable in your community).

Growing your own produce saves you money as does learning to fix things on your own. You will also need to learn to stay fit through natural means, instead of relying on the modern convenience of a gym, as you will need to continue to keep fit even during a disaster so that you can run or fight for your life at any moment's notice. As a result, you can save on a gym membership too.

4. You develop your survival instincts

Performing regular disaster preparedness drills will help you hone your fight-or-flight skills, which come in handy for protecting you in everyday life, for example, helping you avoid accidents or avoid dangerous people.

5. You learn to appreciate nature

Being a prepper means learning to be at one with nature. Our great-grandparents and their great-grandparents survived thanks to nature. Nature has herbs for healing; the wood for fire and warmth and for making survival tools; the berries, fruits, vegetables and mushrooms for energy; the trees for shade, for constructing shelter and hiding from enemies; the rivers for cleaning and bathing; the wildlife for hunting and so on.

It has also been scientifically proven that spending time in nature is great for our mental and emotional health (O'Hare, 2019). The more time you spend in nature learning and honing your survival skills, and building your bug-out location, the more happy and content you will become. This will also benefit other areas of your life, like your work and your relationships.

5 Things To Avoid As A Prepper

1. Relying on your gear instead of your skills

While your gear is important, having the skills to use it correctly during a disaster is even more important. Without your skills, your gear is useless: you may have a gun, but if you don't know how to use it, you won't be able to protect yourself. Likewise, with knowledge of your skills, you still have a good chance of survival because you will know how to build makeshift tools instead. To survive, you will need the following skills:

- Preparing food

- Preparing water

- Combat

- Using weapons and firearms

- Building, preparing, and caretaking an off-grid home.

- First aid and basic medical skills

- Growing food and raising livestock

- Hunting

There are many skills that you will need as a prepper. The best way to gain them all is to go through different scenarios that you may encounter as a prepper and jot down all the skills you will need to survive that scenario.

2. Not being prepared

Imagine this scenario: A disaster has happened and gangs have started looting people's homes. You have a reputation for being a prepper, which means you are in danger. You hear someone coming down your street, so you rush upstairs to get your defensive gear only to find that it is still in its packaging and you do not know how to use it. Make sure you are prepared and know how to use your equipment properly.

It would be ironic to be a prepper and not be prepared on the day of an emergency.

Another tip for being prepared is to read as many books on prepping as you can. What's more, keep the most important ones for use during times of a disaster. For example, you may need to fix a very specific problem with your off-grid waste management system. The information for fixing it may be too niche for you to remember, so having the book on hand during a crisis could become a lifesaver!

3. Inadequate food or water

Be careful not to underestimate how much water and food you will need in survival mode. Humans can typically survive much longer without food. However, you have a maximum of three days without water before you die. So you must be extra careful when prepping to ensure that you are prepped for water supply. As a general rule of thumb, an average person needs two gallons of water per day.

As with all preparation for survival, you want to prep so that you have enough rationed for two weeks. This means that you will need to store a lot of water. Especially if you are on the run, you will need to have a way to purify water.

It's generally best to have a few days of water with you and then the means to purify water as well. That way you have some water to drink while you try to find a source of water if you already do not have one.

Another way to prep for water is to map out areas within your vicinity that have good sources of water, such as rivers and lakes, and use a purification kit. You can then get water from these sources purified and have enough water for survival.

Last, you may want to invest in water-catching devices that can store water from the rain.

When storing food, don't get carried away with only storing the staples like beans and flour. While these are great for energy, you also need a wide source and variety of food to get all your minerals and vitamins in. Store multivitamins to help you power your brain, ward off fatigue, anxiety, and sickness, and cope with stress.

Your body just cannot eat the same food over and over again. Eventually, it will shut down and reject eating the same food. This is why it's important to learn how to grow your own food and even keep livestock, because you're then able to have a wide variety of nutrients from food.

You can stock up on minerals and vitamins because you can then take these once in a while if your body is not willing to eat the food that you have stored or you don't have a food source that contains certain essential vitamins or minerals.

You may also want to map out the surrounding area to note the best sources of berries, edible mushrooms, fish, medicinal plants, and animals. Don't forget to stock up on seasoning herbs, salt, and more because eating food without seasoning is a miserable existence!

If you store large amounts of water, make sure that you're using it within at least three days to avoid contamination and disease. Follow a similar rule for food. Keep a detailed account of when you store food so that you can always eat food with the closest expiration date. This way, you prevent wasting food during a time of disaster when even the smallest bit of food could be the difference between life and death. Likewise, you do not want to eat expired food unknowingly, as you want to avoid being even mildly sick during a disaster/apocalypse.

4. Under-preparing or over-preparing

As a prepper, you can easily fall into the trap of over-preparing for food and water, ignoring other important things that you must prepare for as a result. If you have type 1 diabetes, for example, you need to ensure that you have enough insulin to survive for a few months. You also want to ensure that you prepare for medical emergencies in the form of a first aid kit. Likewise, you want to have adequate ways to start a fire, like matches.

Do you have a torch for an emergency light supply? Do you have an emergency sleeping bag, cooking equipment, blankets, and clothing? Do you have sunscreen and sun-protective clothing? These are all important things you need to take into consideration when prepping to ensure that you are not under-prepared. Even the smallest under-preparation or over-preparation could be the defining factor between life and death; between being saved and being left behind.

You don't want to fall into the trap of over-preparing for self-defense and self-protection. Yes, you need guns and ammo, but you also don't need too many bullets and guns taking up space for the essentials, like medication, food, and water. You also want to be prepared with things that you can barter with in the event of collapse when money becomes valueless. Food, water, and medication are the most valuable currency during a disaster.

Furthermore, even though you will need guns and bullets for hunting, you don't want to have it in your mind that you will easily kill people. You also need to protect your mental health. In fact, you especially need to protect your mental health because this is what will see you through a disaster or collapse. It's no small thing to kill someone, and everyone will be acting out of instinct in a disaster situation. Understand their motive and choose any form of a deterrent rather than fatally injuring someone. If, for example, someone tries to rob you of your food, rather than shooting them, bear spray or a baton will do enough damage.

Practice using different types of knives for hunting, butchering, wood chopping, and self-defense.

Lastly, don't be under-prepared for your pets. If they are city/indoor pets, they will need your help to survive during a disaster. They may not be able to walk long distances, for example, or catch their own food for survival. You must pack for their survival too, including medication, water, first aid, and clothing.

For the sake of your mental health, you must also prepare yourself for the harsh realities of owning a pet when shit hits the fan. Other survivors may target your pet as a good source. If things get really bad, you will have to eat your pet for survival.

5. Being inflexible

Unfortunately, when disaster strikes or when shit hits the fan, we cannot predict how it will unfold. There are so many variables and so many ways for a disaster to occur. That is why you just cannot have an inflexible plan. You might say that you'll meet up with your family at a certain place, but find that your car is no longer working or public transportation has stopped being operational, effective immediately.

This is why being flexible with your plans will give you a better chance of survival. This does not mean that you entirely dismiss having a special place to meet up with your family. Rather, you might have a backup plan where each family member carries an emergency phone with them at all times, so that if shit hits the fan, you're able to communicate with each other to decide on a new place to meet.

With so many ways that disaster can occur, creating as many plans as possible for disaster is a great way to be prepared.

CHECK-IN EXERCISE

Before we proceed with the rest of the book, let's first explore where you are right now in your Off-Grid Journey. This exercise will help you measure how ready you would be to face disaster if it occurred right now. They are designed after each chapter in the book so that you can check in real-time how much your knowledge is increasing as you go through the chapters and what level/skill of prepping you have gained after each chapter.

Below, rate yourself on a scale of 1-5 on how accurate the statements are for you. A score of 1 means "not accurate," and a score of 5 means "very accurate." After you have rated yourself according to the statements, add the total of your scores, then read "What Your Score Really Means" to determine the outcome of your results.

Check-in Statement	Self Rating
I am completely sure that I can live off the grid.	

I have a detailed idea of what it takes to be self-sufficient.	
My bug-out bag contains everything I need to survive for 3 days.	
I know where I will source water and how to purify it.	
I have stored food for emergencies and am now food self-sufficient.	
I have decided whether it is best for me to bug-in or bug-out. I know how to fortify my home for bugging in and how to create my own bunker or shelter for bugging out.	
I have a basic knowledge of first aid to treat either myself or my family.	
I know how to create a basic off-grid waste system.	

I know how to keep myself safe from enemies during a disaster.	
I have an emergency plan for any disaster scenario that could happen right now.	
TOTAL SCORE:	

WHAT YOUR SCORE REALLY MEANS

Score: 10-15

You are not prepared for a disaster and will struggle to keep yourself and your family safe during an emergency.

Don't worry! That's why this book is here. We will go through all the key points that will have you moving from a beginner to an expert.

Score: 16 - 30

You have a basic understanding of what it means to be a prepper, but you should review your strategies and make changes to enhance your preparedness.

Great job! You know the basics, and that is definitely a good start. However, you may need to make some changes to give yourself the best chance of surviving any situation.

Score: 31+

You are almost ready for survival during a disaster! Review your plans to ensure they are ready to go.

KEY CHAPTER TAKEAWAY

You are now on your way to becoming a prepper! You deserve heavy congratulations! To help you out, here are some key takeaways as you think about getting started on your prepping journey.

- A prepper stands tall to take control of their life when society collapses and disaster occurs.

- Being a prepper is simply common sense. You are honoring and following your natural human instinct for survival.

- The preparedness pyramid guides you on which disasters to prep for first and those to prep for last because of their likelihood of happening.

As you go through the next chapters, we would advise that you return to the check-in statements and quiz yourself periodically. Those check-in statements are designed specifically to test your ability to survive in the case of a disaster. We cannot stress enough how disaster often arrives in an instant.

We would love to live in a world where the Earth warns us of a deadly earthquake before it happens, but, alas, we don't! Even when scientists or government officials can give us warnings beforehand, you risk not being able to find an essential supply or not having enough time to learn how to use a weapon for self-defense.

Prepping is a matter of life and death. It is as simple as that. Life is divided into two unique categories: those who die and those who survive. There is no in-between. So, it is better to be safe than sorry. And what better way to do so than by judging your prepping skills at the end of every chapter, and referring to the check-in statements above to see how ready you are to face and survive a disaster if it hits you right now?

In the next chapter, you will learn how to create a bug-out bag (if you don't already have one) as the first step in your emergency response if you need to immediately leave home.

CHAPTER TWO:
BUGGING OUT

What is a bug-out bag? How do you prepare a bug-out bag? Whether you're new to prepping or you're more experienced, you may be wondering how to prepare a bug-out bag and what to put in a bug-out bag.

Even if you already have one, it's always a good idea to refresh your bug-out bag periodically, to ensure that it contains the things that you need to survive, depending on your location, your climate, the people in your survival party, and other outside variables. Quite simply, your bug-out bag is the first step in creating an emergency response to any scenario. This chapter will teach you how to (or, for more seasoned preppers, refresh your memory on how to):

- Identify what a bug-out bag is.

- Learn the benefits of a bug-out bag and why it's useful.

- Make a checklist of what you need in a bug-out bag.

So, we return to the fundamental question: "What is a bug-out bag?" A bug-out bag is essentially a bag made for survival. In this bag, you have all the essential things that you need to survive in a life-or-death scenario. It is meant to be big enough to contain your survival rations and equipment, but also small and light enough to be easy to carry, even in harsh weather and conditions.

So, a bug-out bag will not have your favorite bar of chocolate. It will, however, have things like a flashlight, emergency medication, such as inhalers if you are asthmatic, and water, or the means of purifying dirty water. A bug-out bag is always ready for use in case of an emergency. This means that it is always complete with everything you need and placed in an easy-to-reach position so that you can pick it up and go at any moment. A great way to remember the essential purpose of a bug-out bag is to use the BUG framework:

- *B*e prepared to leave at any minute.

- *Utilize* the "survival rule of 3."

- *G*et only what's necessary for a life-or-death scenario.

Bug-out bags typically have different names, such as the 72-hour-bag. However, their basic function is always the same.

At this point, you may be eager to know what to include in your bug-out bag. But, before we dive into this information, it is important to understand why bug-out bags are so important to have in your home and are ready to go. Why do preppers rely on bug-out bags so much?

Bug-out bags are very versatile. That means that you can prepare for any emergency. If the area in which you live is prone to severe flooding, you can prepare for floods by placing all your important documents in waterproof containers. The trick is to pack essentials that would help *you* survive.

You may not need to pack your prescription reading glasses since you don't use them, while your wife may need to pack her regular glasses since she relies on them for sight. If you live in an area where there are no natural disasters, your bug-out bag will not prepare for that. It might prepare for when *shit hits the fan,* for example, a sudden military coup.

Unfortunately, when disaster hits, time is of the essence. Every single second counts. If the government is evacuating people and you get to the evacuation point even one second too late, that could be the difference between surviving or dying. While the world may want to believe in *Kumbaya* and "positive vibes," the truth is that humans prioritize themselves over each other when in a disaster.

Our brains are designed to keep us alive at all costs—even if that means others perish. Don't be lulled into a false sense of security in case of a disaster or when shit hits the fan. The surrounding people can very easily turn against you since disaster brings about survival-of-the-fittest conditions.

So, how do you become the fittest? Well, one way is to be the fastest. In the wild, the fastest gazelle avoids the lion and can avert disaster. You must do the same. As soon as a disaster hits, you need to prioritize your time. You can't afford to spend two hours packing for everything that you need. You also can't spend an additional 30 minutes looking for one thing or another and not knowing where it is.

Imagine, for example, you are caught up in a fire. In this instance, the one thing that you need is water. If you need to walk or drive away from the fire, you will quickly become fatigued with no water. A good bug-out bag contains water to keep you alive. Remember, the B in B.U.G stands for, "**be** prepared to leave at any minute."

Don't forget that sometimes disasters can force us to stay home. We saw this happen at the beginning of the coronavirus epidemic when we were all forced to stay indoors for long periods. Well, if you're in a lockdown, or otherwise forced to stay indoors for a long time to survive, you will need rations and survival equipment to stay alive.

You may need self-protection as well. Therefore, bug-out bags are not just for venturing out into the wild. They are also for surviving at home. We like to think about our bug-out bags as a way to take our homes with us wherever we are. If you think about it, your home contains things you need to survive on a day-to-day basis, from water to food to tools and even self-protective gear.

The bug-out bag is just a way of making your home mobile. Consequently, you find that you can use many things that you already have at home when you're trying to create your bug-out bag.

Last, bug-out bags are actually an excellent way to practice minimalism. Go into any of your neighbors' houses and you will find it filled with junk they don't need. Preppers are, by nature, anti-consumption because we know that food, water and medicine are so much more important than a new pair of designer sneakers. Without fail, we prioritize our survival, preferring to focus on what is essential in life—not what is popular.

The more you prep your bug-out bag and help others prep theirs, the more skilled you become at learning how to determine if an item is essential or not—both in everyday life and during times of disaster.

What Needs To Go In It?

Your bug-out bag must be created based on the survival rule of 3. The survival rule of 3 states that there are 3 things that you cannot survive without. They are: food, water, and air. As a result, the first things you pack into your bug-out bag should meet these needs.

Food

You can survive **3 weeks** without food.

3 weeks of food is too much to carry. In addition, your bug-out bag is purposed to help you survive the first 72 hours of a disaster, so pack enough food for 3 days. Those three days' worth of food will give you enough energy to seek out alternative sources of fresh food, whether it be through foraging, hunting, or fishing. Therefore, ensure that you pack calorie-dense, protein-dense, and carb-dense food that can keep you energized for a long time.

You should also pack foods that contain essential micro-nutrients, such as vitamins and minerals. Without the macronutrients found in fruit and vegetables, your body will begin to deteriorate fast.

Water

You can survive **3 days** without water before you die.

Unfortunately, water is very heavy. Even carrying a 3-liter bottle will get heavy very soon. Adding a water purification system will help you purify the water on the go. You can purify water from off-grid sources like rainwater, streams, and lakes, as well as from on-grid sources, like tap water. You should also carry a water bottle or bladder that can be easily collapsed when empty, for easy, space-saving storage. Whenever you find water, you can fill up your bottle/bladder.

Air

You can survive **3 minutes** without oxygen.

You will need a handy way to purify your air in case the air becomes badly polluted, so an air filtration mask is paramount to our survival.

Other essentials you need in your bug-out bag (not based on the survival rule of 3) are:

Shelter

You can survive only **3 hours** in a harsh environment without shelter. Harsh environments include things like freezing climates, hot weather, floods, storms and more.

You will need to pack a sleeping bag, tent, space blanket, and any other items needed to create a temporary shelter.

Clothing

Perhaps clothing is just an offshoot of shelter, i.e. a way to protect your skin and body from damaging elements. Don't pack just the basics. A shirt, trousers and a jacket might seem to be common sense, but you will also use your hands a lot in a survival situation.

Remember that humans evolved to use our hands as tools and weapons. We survived because we have dexterous fingers to accomplish complicated tasks. Hence, you want to protect your hands because they are your greatest tool for survival during a disaster. Use gloves while working, for example, while chopping wood or gathering firewood. Likewise, use gloves to protect your hands in case it gets really cold. You do not want to get frostbite on your fingers, as this will lead to serious health complications.

Likewise, protect your head from the cold with headgear-like caps and keep a change of clothes to prevent discomfort and even hypothermia from wearing damp clothes.

Heat/Warmth

The easiest way to provide heat and warmth is to start a fire. While you can easily find wood or other materials to start a fire. The problem is finding a spark. So, carry matches and other types of fire starters that can be stored safely in your bug-out bag.

If you have space, put hand warmers and foot warmers in your bug-out bag. They would be very useful in keeping you warm in freezing climates. Of course, in tropical climates, pack clothes that would enable you to regulate your body temperature. You may want to pack UV protective clothing to keep you protected from the harmful effects of UV radiation.

Power Source

You will want to keep in touch with family members, friends, and emergency services while on the move. You will also want to keep in contact with those around you to improve your chances of survival. Phone batteries run out and solar chargers won't be as effective if there is no sunlight. A fully charged, high Mah Power-Bank will provide an emergency source of electricity for charging all your other bug-out devices.

Lighting

You need light to function at night. Electricity is more than likely guaranteed to fail in a disaster, even if only temporarily. You will need light at night to carry out basic functions like cooking and using the toilet. You will also need it to protect yourself from predators and from other humans who may want to harm you.

A source of light will also enable rescue searchers to find you much easier. Chemlights, headlights, and flashlights are significant sources of light. We recommend you purchase a solar charger for your lighting sources so you can charge them on the go. Pack spare batteries as additional backups.

Defense

You want a very reliable and sturdy knife for your bug-out bag. It will come in very handy when trying to cut/chop wood for fire or to even harvest plants and crops. It can also be used as a self-defense weapon against animals and other attackers. Make sure that your knife is in a sheath so that you don't harm yourself or others accidentally.

You should always also carry pepper spray because it is a great way to disarm animals and humans without resorting to bloodshed. Remember that you don't want to kill unless it is absolutely necessary.

Finally, there are always other items that you can use as a weapon in your bug-out bag. Anything can be a weapon. You may be walking and see a large, heavy stick. This in itself can be a suitable weapon for you to use to stun attackers. Always keep your eye out for anything that can be used as a weapon and keep it as close by as possible.

First Aid

Your first aid kit should have the essential items needed for a first aid kit, including additional items like sunscreen. It should also come with first aid instructions, since you may not be familiar with how to use certain items. The checklist below will list all the first aid items you need.

Navigation Tools

A good GPS system, map of the area, and compass are all very good survival items to carry with you. Even if you might think you know the area very well, you can still get lost and stuck, unable to find your way out of an area.

Multi-purpose Tools

Multi-purpose tools can be used to dig, build and secure shelter, chop wood, hunt, fish, create traps, protect yourself, make repairs, break tough things, clear paths, and carry out other actions that you need to survive.

Miscellaneous

Miscellaneous things include radios (to keep in contact with the world around you), walkie-talkies (for communication), copies of important documents, your passport, sewing kits, contact details and addresses of loved ones, goggles (to protect your eyes), ear muffs or ear plugs (to protect your ears) and so on.

BUG-OUT BAGS ON A BUDGET

Even if you are on a tight budget, there are still ways to make a cheap bug-out bag for each member of your family. Remember that there is no need to go out and buy new things if you already have them in your home! Rummage around and see what you can find to save money. This way, you can create your bug-out bag for under $20.

Ensure the bag you purchase is thick, durable, and strong. You don't want the straps to break while you are running from gunfire, for instance. Try to purchase a good one on sale to stay within your budget. Ensure it is water-resistant and air-tight; has padded, thick straps; separated pockets, with many compartments; and roll-top expanded storage.

BUDGET BUG-OUT BAG CHECKLIST

Here is what you should pack in your bug-out bag on a budget:

- Durable backpack
- Band-aids
- Alcohol wipes
- Bottle(s) of water
- Chargeable flashlight
- Pen and notepad
- Snack bars and energy/protein bars
- Cash
- Emergency blanket
- Change of clothes, underwear, and socks
- Toothbrush and toothpaste
- Thick beach towel
- Map of local area
- Dust mask/bandana
- Prescription medication
- Spare prescription glasses
- Alcohol wipes
- Pocket knife
- Chap-Stick
- Soap
- Deodorant
- Work gloves/leather gloves
- Deck of cards, palm-sized games and/or a book
- Charging cable(s)

- Ziplock bags
- Poncho or umbrella
- Fork and spoon

- USB wall plugs
- Durable plastic cup
- Lighter/matches

AN IDEAL CHECKLIST

The items in your bug-out bag may vary slightly based on your specific needs and your location. Nonetheless, the essentials that you need will not change. You may think, for example, that you do not need a warm jacket in a hot climate, but temperatures could fall dramatically at night, leaving you at risk if you cannot protect yourself. Below is an ideal bug-out bag checklist to help you pack, for when SHTF or when disaster strikes.

- Air filtration mask
- Water carrying solution
- Sunscreen
- Painkillers
- Ax
- Duct tape
- Multi-tool
- Anti-bacterial antiseptic wipes

- Water filtration system
- Emergency food rations
- Bandages/band-aids
- Mini-shovel
- Crowbar
- Foldable saw
- Paracord
&
- Antibiotic ointment

- First aid kit (with instructions)
- Gauze pads
- Medical gloves
- Burn gel
- Sling
- Tourniquet
- Sleeping bag
- Tent
- Space blanket
- Air filtration mask
- Fishing kit
- Waterproof jacket
- Change of clothes, including underwear and socks
- Cold weather gloves
- Fingerless heavy-duty gloves
- Hand warmers
- Headgear
- Headlamp
- Change of clothes
- Knife
- Pepper spray
- Whistle
- Hand warmers
- Matches, lighter, or other suitable fire starter
- Chemlights
- Flashlights
- Compass
- Maps of your local area
- GPS tracking system
- Charger
- Goggles
- Sewing kit

- Copies of important documents in two USB sticks
- Prescription drugs
- Power source
- Goggles
- Emergency cash
- Small mirror
- Ear muffs/plugs

Although this is an ideal list, it is better to have a more limited bug-out bag than no bag at all. Half a loaf is better than none, meaning that it is better to use what you have now and at least create something that will last you a few days in a worst-case scenario than to have nothing at all.

BUG-OUT PLAN

Along with your bug-out bag, you will also need a bug-out plan. Your bug-out plan is even more important than your bug-out bag because you can survive without a bug-out bag as long as you have a plan. During a disaster, it is very difficult to think about what you need to do and how to do it well to survive. Your body is running on adrenaline and you are not clear of mind. A bug-out plan essentially prevents you from making mistakes but helps you to make the best decisions that ensure survival.

Here are five steps you need to consider when making a bug-out plan:

1. **What kind of disasters are most likely to occur in your area?**

What natural disasters typically occur in your area, such as earthquakes or floods? What other types of disasters have your area suffered from? You can't prepare for every disaster, so knowing the most likely disaster you will face in your area helps you tailor your bug-out plan for the best chance of survival.

2. **What strengths and weaknesses are you working with or against?**

If you are the strongest one in the family, perhaps you will carry the baby if you have to walk long distances. If you have a doctor in the family, they will be in charge of every medical emergency. Your bug-out plan should complement your strengths and prepare for your weaknesses. If you don't know how to read maps and compasses or identify which local plants are edible or poisonous, your bug-out plan tells you how to do this.

The more skills you gain before disaster strikes, the less you have to carry in your bag. For example, you may not need to carry much food if you know where to find food in your local forest.. For example, you may not need to carry much food if you know where to find food in your local forest.

3. Plan for specific destinations.

Where exactly do you want to be when disaster strikes? Also, where do you and your family, friends, neighbors, or any other members of your survival group want to meet? You could all be at separate places when disaster strikes. So deciding where to meet is a great bug-out plan.

Another reason to have a specific location is that you can keep other survival materials there. This also means that you don't have to carry as much in your bug-out bag. It also gives you great peace of mind to know that there is a destination waiting for you: there is a home waiting for you. A positive mindset increases your chances of survival.

Great locations to meet are your relatives' house, your second home or your cabin. You can also meet at large public facilities or local shelters.

4. Plan for four destinations.

Your plan is to get to a safe destination in the event of a disaster. However, your safe destination might not be safe after all. Perhaps it has experienced the same disaster that you have. Or, perhaps, refugees are not being allowed in. It is best to practice having four destinations, at least, as part of your bug-out plan. Make sure that there is a destination on each cardinal direction on the map, i.e. North, South, East, West. This keeps your plans flexible in case of any unforeseen circumstances.

5. Calculate your average travel speed.

How long would it take you to reach your destination? To find this out you will need to calculate your average travel speed. This will let you know how much you can carry with you. You don't want to carry a bug-out bag with all the essentials, only to find that you cannot carry it after a certain time because it is too heavy. Typically, you will only be able to carry a bag that weighs 25% of your weight. You will carry your bag for hours and days. Ensure it is not too heavy.

Usually, the average person can walk 2.5-4 miles per hour on flat terrain. If there are children, pets, or vulnerable people in your party, this will take, at least, twice as long. Additionally, the terrain in your local area will give you an idea of how fast you can walk. If it is downhill or uphill, you, of course, will need more time than average.

GET HOME BAG

Any good prepper in the know has a get-home bag (GHB). Your get-home bag, as the name suggests, helps you get home after a disaster. Your goal is to get home as quickly as possible. Perhaps you were at work when disaster struck and need to get home to pick up your kids and your bug-out bag. Or perhaps you need to get home to pick up your pets.

You use a get-home bag when you are not too far away from home. Obviously, you will not choose to use a get home back if you were in Australia and your home is in Alaska. As a result, your GBH should be light and keep you alive for no more than a couple of days. You need to pack only the very basic essentials, like a water bottle and water filter, and food to keep you going, such as trail mix and energy bars. You may also pack a few other tool basics, such as a multi-tool, duct tape, and a first aid kit. Keep your GHB where you spend the most time outside of the home. This would be in your workplace or in your car. For children, this will be in their lockers at school.

SURVIVAL TASK

Think about the five most important items that you will need in your bug-out bag. This could be important medication, contact details, prescription glasses, and so many other items. Make sure these five items can meet your personal needs. The aim is to personalize your bug-out bag to your own needs, too. Your five items should also be items found in at least one checklist in this book.

Key Chapter Takeaway

- Refresh your bug-out bag periodically, ensuring it contains all you need to survive in a life-or-death scenario.

- Bug-out bags are not just for venturing out into the wild. They are also for surviving at home.

- A bug-out bag is always ready for use in case of an emergency.

- The items in your bug-out bag may vary slightly based on your specific needs and your location.

- Your bug-out bag must be created based on the survival rule of 3. The survival rule of 3 states that there are 3 things that you cannot survive without food, water, and air.

- It is better to have a more limited bug-out bag than no bag at all.

- Your bug-out plan is even more important than your bug-out bag because you can survive without a bug-out bag as long as you have a plan.

In the next chapter, you will learn how to store an emergency supply of water, how to purify water, and how to find a source of water once those supplies have run out.

Chapter Three:
Hydration Is Key

You can go 3 days without water before you die. This doesn't seem like a big deal when you have running water coming out of every faucet in your house, but life can be very precarious, as are the systems and infrastructure we have in place to keep us alive. All it takes is one storm or one burst pipe and you could suddenly find yourself without water to drink or with only contaminated water available. Once that happens, the clock is ticking down for you and your family.

For many non-preppers, this will be a difficult life-or-death situation. For you, this will be another challenge you wisely prepped for. The cold, hard fact of life is that being thirsty is a horrible feeling. Our ancestors knew this, and that is why they always stored clean, drinkable, non-contaminated water.

Like our ancestors, your goal is to keep even more water than you need to increase your chances of survival. As any good prepper would surmise, hydration is, indeed, key. To prep you for staying hydrated during a disaster, remember the framework, W.A.S.P.S.

- **W**hen in doubt, double your ration.

- **A**lways drink now and worry about later.

- **S**anitize containers to stay alive.

- **P**urify your water without fail.

- **S**ource your water from many sources!

We have become too used to having running water, but it takes just one disaster to snap us out of our spoiled state. As a serious prepper, here are the water facts you need to memorize to face disaster head-on:

- How much do you need to store?

- How to store it.

- How to source clean water.

- How to purify water.

HOW MUCH WATER SHOULD I STORE?

The standard storage unit for water is one gallon per day per person. Usually, a regularly active person will need to drink about half a gallon of water daily, but doubling it errs on the side of caution. You will need water not just for drinking but also for cooking and cleaning, so you will need to double it if you plan to do more than drinking it. Remember, when in doubt, double your ration.

How much water you decide to store depends on your needs. Do you plan to be on the move? In that case, you cannot carry with you 30 gallons of water. A water purifier on the go would be your best choice. However, if you plan to survive in a bunker or another such location, then storing as much water as your storage would allow is a good idea. You will also need to think about where/how to store water, as will be discussed later in this chapter.

No matter what happens, do not ration water. Always drink now and worry about water later. Drink however much water you need to survive for the day and then try to find more water the next day. Rationing water is like trying to ration oxygen—it just won't work. You can try to reduce your need for water, however, by keeping cool and reducing your level of activity. Keep in mind the survival rule of 3. You need food, water, and air. Water and air are the topmost important priority for any human. No other need can be fulfilled unless those two are prioritized.

HOW TO STORE WATER

The number one rule for storing water is to store it in a cool, dry place, e.g. a pantry or a basement. This will prevent bacteria and other microorganisms from growing and contaminating your water. The easiest way to store water is in a reusable container with a lid and one that is easy to carry. This makes empty water bottles, bricks, canisters, and barrels a great resource for storing water. To save on space, you can purchase collapsible bottles and canisters that take up less space when empty and are easy to carry while on the move.

Pre-bottled water will typically last 2-5 years if left unopened, making it a great way to store water. It is also affordable, portable, easy to carry, and widely available. Bigger storage containers, like 5-gallon water containers, are an alternative water storage method for storing larger quantities of water. You can also purchase 55-gallon water barrels for your bug-out shelter. If used well, a barrel can last one person for a month. If you want to store even more water in one go (following the framework of doubling your ration), purchase 160-gallon water storage tanks or a Water Bob, which is a device that allows you to fill up your tub with water without contaminating the water with your well-used tub.

You will need to replace your pre-bottled water once it expires, to prevent contamination. For alternative water storage options, use food-grade, non-degradable, sanitized, airtight containers that have never been used to store a hazardous substance. In a pinch, you can also use other containers in your home, as long as you sanitize them and they have not been previously used to store hazardous materials.

How to Source Water

It might seem like the pressure to source water is enormous, but there are always options, unless, of course, you decide to bug out in the Sahara desert. Even then, there are oases in the desert for sourcing water. There will always be a source of water. Simply put, your chances of survival increase the more sources you use. That way, when one method fails (whether temporarily or permanently) there is another to keep you alive.

Your three primary sources of emergency water supply are:

1. Emergency water sources inside your home.

There are some excellent sources of emergency water in your home. They are:

Ice

If you have a freezer, then you have ice. You never know when your electricity will go out or come back on during a disaster, so it is a good idea to empty your freezer (and fridge) as quickly as possible. Otherwise, you might find yourself looking at spoiled food, as well as a defrosted freezer making a messy puddle around your kitchen.

To collect ice from your freezer, simply scrape the ice into a bowl and allow it to defrost for a few minutes or hours. If you don't need to use the ice right away, you can put the bowl back into the freezer, still containing the ice. That way it can continue to keep your food preserved for at least a few hours until you're ready to use the ice or eat the food.

Shelf-Stable Beverages

Shelf stable beverages are beverages that can last a long time when left unopened. Things like fruit juices and cartons of milk are significant sources of water since they contain nutrients and electrolytes that your body desperately needs.

You will of course still need to drink water, however, they can act as a short-term replacement once or twice a day.

Don't be fooled into thinking that carbonated beverages can be a great water replacement source. Along with alcoholic beverages and caffeinated drinks, they actually deplete your body of water, leaving you even more dehydrated than if you have not drunk them in the first place. You certainly don't want to be dehydrated in a disaster scenario because it can quickly turn dangerous if you cannot find water on time.

Household Pipes

Even after the main water supply is turned off in your home, there is still water stored in the pipes. You can't turn on the taps to get the water, so you will need to use gravity. To do this, you need to turn on the lowest level faucet in your house to the highest level. This pumps air into your plumbing and causes a steady drip of water to trickle out. Since it is normal water from your pipes, it is drinkable for the next few days.

Hot Water Heater/Tank

Hot water heaters/tanks are like your pipes. They always have water stored in them. Depending on the hot water heater you have, it will have between 20-50 gallons of water stored in it. This water is, of course, the same as the water in your pipes, which is then fed into your water heater. So this means that it is clean and drinkable. Make sure you shut off the main water valve immediately before or after a disaster (whichever you can manage) to prevent contamination.

We've already mentioned water heaters are all very different. As is the creed of every prepper, you must be prepared. In the case of your water heater, this means knowing what type and grade of water heater you have.

Become familiar with it to understand its design and how it works. Unlike a non-prepper, you will be prepared with all the information and tools you need to work your water heater efficiently when disaster strikes. Frankly, it is impossible to read a water heater manual when a tornado is approaching, for example. To get the water stored in your hot water tank/heater, follow the instructions below:

1. Read your hot water tank manual to familiarize yourself with how your tank works.

2. Turn off the electric or gas supply to your hot water heater. If it is a natural gas heater, you will need to turn the handle perpendicular to the pipe to turn it off.

3. Turn off the water intake valve located at the top of your water heater. Turning it off will protect the water stored in your heater from contamination.

4. Find the pressure and temperature relief valve found either at the top or side of your tank.

5. Protect the water in the tank from outside contamination by turning off the water intake valve at the top of the tank. This will allow the water to flow by breaking suction. You will not need to shut off your intake valve or power source if you are only planning

on collecting a few gallons of water as part of your regular practice.

6. Use a handy tool, such as a screwdriver, to turn on the drain valve faucet. The drain valve faucet is located at the bottom of the tank/heater. Use a clean, non-contaminated container to collect the water.

7. You and everyone else in your survival party should follow these steps to practice draining water from your hot water tank regularly. The good news is that draining water from your tank regularly will prolong the life of your water heater by removing sediment and particles that build up at the bottom.

You can already see that there are good places inside your home to find emergency water sources. As a prepper, being able to see things that other non-preppers cannot see is what distinguishes you from those who may not survive. This is an impressive skill to develop because, no matter where you find yourself during a disaster, you need to be able to spot emergency water sources to survive.

2. Emergency water sources around your home.

Just like emergency water sources inside your home, there are many sources of emergency water around your home. Some of the best ones are:

Rainwater

Did you know that in many countries today rainwater is still collected as a source of free clean water? And why not? Rainwater has always been collected by humans because it is nature's way of providing us with good, uncontaminated water.

Depending on where you are in the world collecting rainwater might be illegal so, we would recommend that you look up laws in your area and country. During a disaster, you won't be prosecuted for collecting rainwater to survive.

You can create your own makeshift rainwater catchment system using your rain gutters and a clean rain barrel. If you don't have a rain barrel, a clean large container or bucket will also work fine. Rainwater is generally clean unless it comes into contact with a dirty surface or with the ground. If this occurs, filter and purify your water with the methods described in this chapter.

Swimming Pool

Swimming pool water may not seem like an obvious choice of clean water, especially for drinking, however it is entirely doable if the water is treated and has not been swum in. Don't drink it, but it is still an excellent source of hygienic water, for example, water for taking a shower or cleaning your home.

You will need, however, to filter your swimming pool water as it will contain chemicals such as chlorine. By distilling the water, you make it safe to drink and use. Distilling the water basically removes all the impurities and chemicals from it. You might be tempted to think that boiling swimming water is good enough to make it clean and pure, however, this will not remove chemicals already in the water. You can harm yourself if you drink boiled swimming pool water, so be careful!

The Big Berkey Water Filter (described below) is great for distilling swimming pool water and claims to remove 99.9% of heavy metals and up to 99.9% of chlorine in swimming pool water (Berkey Filters, 2022). Note, however, that they advise you to only use it in emergencies because it significantly decreases the number of uses left on your filter once you filter out swimming pool water (Berkey Filters, 2022). You also have the option to use AquaRain filters to purify swimming pool water. The one downside to these filters is that they do not remove salt or any naturally occurring minerals from the water. Conversely, they are very handy because all you need to do is add AquaRain into a 5-gallon bucket of swimming pool water and it filters it for you!

If you want to use any other brands of filters, that is perfectly fine. You just need to ensure that you do proper research first. Many filter brands may claim to filter and purify water perfectly, but they may not filter out chlorine, salt, minerals, or any other chemicals. It is always a good bet to invest in the more expensive filters because they are more effective.

Plant Transpiration

This method of collecting water will only get you about half a cup of water in five hours. It is not a very effective method of collecting water in general disaster scenarios, but it is a great method for serious emergencies when you have no other alternatives. When plants transpire, they release vapor through their pores. You can collect this water for drinking purposes.

To do so, wrap a clean and sanitized plastic bag around the branch of a living bush or tree. Make sure the branch is in direct sunlight and the plastic bag is not wrapped too tightly. It should have enough space to collect between ⅓ to ½ cup of water. Leave the plastic bag for about 4 to 5 hours, allowing the plant to transpire and release vapor, which the bag will then collect.

Before a disaster occurs, do your research on which plants are toxic. That way, you do not collect toxic water that could cause serious harm to your health. You also have to keep with you, at all times, clean plastic bags that you can use to collect water through transpiration. Memorize how this method works because it is a great emergency water supply while bugging out.

Below-Ground Solar Still

A below-ground solar still uses the same method of collecting water as plant transpiration. How does it work?

Get a clean, sanitized bowl and dig a hole in the ground just big enough to fit this bowl and hold your plant. Make sure the hole is in an area that receives plenty of sunlight for hours at a time. Build a reservoir inside the pit just big enough to hold your bowl, then place your non-toxic plant in the pit.

Use a sheet of clear sanitized plastic to cover the pit and then secure the edges well so that the plastic does not move. You can place stones or other heavy objects around the edges to do this. Then, create an indent in the center of the plastic by placing a rock or slightly heavy object just on top of the position of the bowl in the pit. Don't use an object that is too heavy because it will break the sheet. As the plant transpires, the condensation will rise and build up on the plastic sheet. The indent in the sheet will work with gravity to pull the water downwards into the bowl at the bottom of the pit.

Water Generating Units

A water-generating unit can be used as a backup source of water. Why is it only a backup source of water? Well, it only works with electricity. That means that you cannot use it if the power goes out during a disaster. Nonetheless, following the framework, "source your water from many sources", having one as a backup is never a bad idea!

A water generating unit works by harvesting water in the air and converting it into drinkable water. It works best if you live in a hot and humid climate where there is plenty of condensed moisture in the air to harvest.

3. Emergency water sources from surrounding areas.

Luckily, when a disaster occurs, there are always people around to help. Disaster does not stop every resource from the area from working at the same time, so you will be able to find other sources of water in your surroundings. Simply make sure that the water that you collect from surrounding areas is from clean, uncontaminated sources. Do your due diligence. Ask questions and inspect the sources if you can. Then, filter the water after it is collected.

Some significant sources of emergency water from surrounding areas are:

Local Bodies of Water

There are different types of bodies of water and some are better than others. Flowing water, like rivers, is always better than stagnant water, like lakes. However, the best local body of water source is spring water from an underground source. They are usually the safest water for drinking. Rivers and flowing streams are also often good sources of clean water. You always have to consider the source of the water, as we've already discussed. What is in the surroundings of the underground source of your spring water? What is upstream of your flowing stream or river? This does not mean that you should not filter all sources of water from local bodies even if the source is clean. There are so many ways for pollutants, waste, pesticides, fertilizers, and many other poisonous chemicals to get into local bodies of water, so always take precaution. Remember to always "purify your water without fail."

Stagnant water such as lakes and ponds, on the other hand, is more likely to be contaminated with pollutants. Floodwaters, marshes and swamp water are all severely contaminated and should be avoided even in severe emergencies, unless you have the Big Berkey Water Filter.

Private Well Water

If you or someone in your surrounding area has a well, then this is another good source of emergency water for you. Be cautious because well water can be polluted or contaminated, for example, if a dead animal has fallen into it. Follow the hydration framework and purify it before using.

You will also need a way to get the water out of the well. If the well is not too deep, you can use a hand crank and bucket or a rope tied to a small bucket to get water out. This is a very labor-intensive process, so a pump might be more suitable. While electric pumps are handy, non-electric ones will work even when the electricity is out. There are also solar-powered pumps that you can invest in now if you do indeed have access to a well. While it might seem frivolous to spend money on a solar-powered pump now, it could be a lifesaver when the chips are down. Last, if you have a back-up generator and some fuel, you can use this to pump water.

Water From Government or Humanitarian Agencies

After a disaster, relief efforts are always organized to get to survivors and those in need. Clean, drinkable water is one of the first supplies sent, so chances are that you will receive water from the government and other humanitarian agencies.

Yes, this is always good as a back-up plan, but it is not advisable to rely on this source of water. You will have to stand in line for hours with very cranky, hungry, tired, and desperate people. Things can go south very quickly in such an environment, hence being self-reliant for water is a better choice after all.

WATER PURIFICATION

Even if you're not able to store water, it is imperative that you're able to purify water. If you don't have any stored water, as long as you're able to purify your water, you can go out searching for a source of water. Additionally, in case of emergencies when you need to be on the move, you won't be able to carry water with you because it is very heavy.

A purifier is a perfect in-between option. It is light enough to carry and still provides you with clean water. The only difference is you will need to then source water. Luckily, there are different methods for purifying water depending on which works best for you.

1. Boiling water

Boiling water is the most traditional way of purifying water. Simply boil for ten minutes to allow enough time to kill all the dangerous microorganisms.

2. Iodine

You can use iodine tincture from a first aid kit to purify water if you have no other options. You will need to prep it first: Let it sit for 30 minutes if it's warm outside and an hour if it's hot. Add ten drops per gallon. Don't use too much, otherwise, it can be poisonous.

3. Rocks, sand, and charcoal

This method of purification reduces the bacteria in water and makes it better, although it will not protect you from Giardia. To purify, layer a clean sock (or any other straining container) with sand placed at the bottom. Layer charcoal on the sand then add rocks lastly. Filter your water into a container.

4. Chlorination

Chlorination kills most microorganisms in water. To chlorinate water, there are three methods that you can use. They are:

Chlorine dioxide tablets and water drops

This works by simply dropping the chlorine dioxide tablets into your water and letting the tablets do their job. The tablets treat the water with chemicals that are safe to ingest, killing all the disease-causing microorganisms in the water. You can use portable tablets which work effectively well against bacteria, viruses, Lamblia, Giardia, and Cryptosporidium. You may also use water drops. Ensure that the water drops you choose are EPA-registered. Water drops can chlorinate gallons of water in one go since they are essentially chlorine dioxide tablets in liquid form.

Chlorine bleach

Like chlorine dioxide water drops, chlorine bleach can treat gallons of water in one go with just a little amount. If you decide to use chlorine bleach, you will need to shake the water and then wait for 30 minutes before using it. At the same time, be aware that chlorine bleach does not kill Giardia, as chlorine tablets or drops do. However, it will prevent cholera.

Using bleach to purify water typically follows more rules than using tablets or drops.

First, avoid scented bleaches, bleaches with added cleaners or color-safe bleaches. These types of bleaches are toxic for you and your family, thanks to the added chemicals! They will only contaminate your water. If the bleach contains any types of dyes, perfumes, or other additives, then skip it!

Second, use bleach specifically designed for drinking water and not pool water. Chlorine bleach designed for pool water is a different chemical compound altogether and is a corrosive pesticide. Not only will your water taste bad, but it will also be too toxic for ingestion.

Third, be aware that chlorine bleach is effective for only six months after it is manufactured, so you will need to rotate it often, as well as ensure that you are not using expired bleach.

The simple fact is that bleach is not meant for human consumption. We recommend you keep it only for emergency usage. Why? Well, bleach is carcinogenic. When you add bleach to your water, it oxidizes any organic contaminants living in the water. This process produces trihalomethanes, which are famous for causing cancer.

It is also very important that you follow the instructions on the warning very closely. If you add too much bleach into your water, it will become extremely poisonous and corrosive, also damaging anything it comes in contact with, including your skin, organs, and other body parts.

Therefore, think of bleach as only a short-term option to tide you over until you can find other sources of purifying your water during a disaster.

5. Filtration

Filtering water is a great way to purify it of all disease-causing parasites and any other contaminants. We recommend three different water filters:

Lifestraw Water Filter

As its name suggests, Lifestraw water filter works like a drinking straw that filters water as you drink. It is a lightweight and portable option that filters out 99.9999% of waterborne protozoan parasites and bacteria. It is a great option to place in your bug-out bag for when you are on the move.

Katadyn Water Filter

Used by the military, the Katadyn water filter is a very durable and long-lasting option for filtering up to 13,000 gallons of water with an output of about 1 quart or 1 liter per minute.

Big Berkey Water Filter

The Big Berkey water filter can filter up to 3,000 gallons of water. It is great for everyday use since it is portable, has a long filter life, and can filter not just treated water, but untreated water from stagnant and flowing bodies of water, such as lakes, ponds, and streams.

SURVIVAL TASK

Think where you could store water on your property. What systems do you have in place to purify water? Where is your closest natural water source?

Create a mini-plan containing the information you'll need should water sourcing become a problem during an emergency.

Key Chapter Takeaway

- The standard storage unit for water is one gallon per day per person. You will need to double this to factor in using water for hygiene.

- How much water you decide to store depends on your needs. Will you be on the move or will you be planning on bugging out or bugging in?

- Never ration water. Always drink now and worry about water later.

- Store water in a cool, dry place, preferably with a lid on.

- Pre-bottled bottles of water, bricks, canisters, and barrels are a great resource for storing water.

- Pre-bottled water will typically last 2-5 years if left unopened, making it a great way to store water.

- Replace your pre-bottled water once they expire, to prevent contamination.

- Water storage: use food-grade, non-degradable, sanitized, airtight containers that have never been used to store a hazardous substance.

- There are sources of emergency water in and around your home and in your surrounding area.

- If you're not able to store water, you must be able to purify water. That way, you can go out searching for a source of water.

- Water purifiers help you purify water when you are bugging out.

- There are different methods for purifying water depending on which works best for your situation.

In the next chapter, you will learn the different ways you can store food for emergencies, including the different ways you can become more self-sufficient when thinking long-term about food resources.

CHAPTER FOUR:
CALORIES ARE GOOD!

In an emergency, calories are good. Most of us spend every waking minute counting our calories because we want to eat fewer calories. Ironically, during a disaster, the opposite is true: you want to consume as many calories as you possibly can to stay alive. It is simple human biology: when food is plentiful; you try to eat less. And when food is scarce, you spend your energy and time trying to eat as much as you can.

During a disaster, your nervous system is also working overtime to keep you grounded despite being in a very stressful situation. As a result, your body will seriously rely on calories to keep you working at your most efficient level. Hence, calories become massively important when trying to survive during a disaster.

This chapter aims to explore the different ways that you can store food for emergencies, how much food you should have ready, and also ways you can become more self-sufficient when thinking long-term about food resources.

Yes, you want to store as many calories as you can, but you also want to store them well. Avoiding food contamination and spoilage is just as important as storing the food in the first place. There is just no point going through all of that effort and time, and spending all of that money, stockpiling food, only to have it go to waste because you did not store it properly.

Four types of food contamination can leave you severely sick and even lead to death. They are:

Microbial

Microbial contamination occurs when living microbes in the air contaminate your food. Microbes, such as viruses, fungi, bacteria, mold, and toxins, are toxic to humans. Indeed, microbial contamination is one of the most common causes of food contamination, as well as food poisoning, for humans.

The simple fact is that microbes are everywhere, so you have to take very careful precautions to avoid food contamination. The first thing you must do is ensure that you prepare all your food properly, especially highly contaminable foods like raw chicken and fish. Never eat highly contaminable foods that are not cooked thoroughly, no matter how hungry you are. It is best to stay hungry and forage for food the next day than to eat food that will leave you dead in the next few days.

Another way to prevent microbial contamination is to store and prepare foods that are risky away from other foods. Keep them very separate from your other foods and wash and disinfect all surfaces that they touch as soon as preparation is completed. In fact, clean and disinfect all surfaces in your bug-out residence regularly. This may be difficult when there is not much water, so store bottles of antibacterial spray as a precaution.

Always wash raw fruits and vegetables and take very good care of your hygiene. Wash or disinfect your hands regularly, take regular showers and wash your hair often.

Do not leave out open containers of raw or cooked food at any point because it attracts microbes. Microbes also love moist, humid conditions, so take care to prevent this wherever you store your food. Open windows when it is hot and close them when it is cold and/or humid. Finally, keep all your food in moisture-proof and air-proof containers.

Physical

This physical contamination is any physical object that contaminates your food during the food preparation or storing process. Anything counts as a physical contaminant, including hair, broken glass, stones, fingernails, toys, bits of plastic, jewelry, pests–anything really. Not only can physical contamination cause things like choking or broken teeth, it can also carry microbes that end up causing food poisoning.

You can prevent physical food contamination by keeping all your foods in tight and sealed containers. Don't use damaged cooking or food storage equipment that can break into your food, remove all jewelry and pull back your hair before cooking. Last, cultivate an environment that is unfriendly to pests. Keep your food storage and preparation area clean and dry at all times and keep it at cool temperatures to dissuade pests. Make sure there are no openings for pests to enter your food storage areas, such as windows and chimneys, and fumigate regularly. To cultivate an area unfriendly to pests, never leave cooked or raw food out for even short periods. The smell alone is enough to attract them.

Allergenic

We all know what allergies are and we all know how serious they can get. Even if no one in your survival party is allergic to anything, don't forget that allergies can start at any time in a person's life, so always store allergenic-free food, just in case.

If there is a person with allergies in your survival party, then you must always keep allergenic food separate from all your other food and avoid using the same kitchen utensils, preparation area, and clothes for all these. Clean and disinfect your kitchen often, as we've already discussed, and stick to food that comes from suppliers who take allergenic contamination seriously.

There are 14 major food allergies. They are:

1. Milk

2. Eggs

3. Celery and celeriac (found in stock cubes, ready meals, spice mixes, sauces, and savory flavorings)

4. Fish

5. Sesame seeds

6. Crustacean shellfish

7. Tree nuts

8. Sulfur dioxide and sulfite (found in dehydrated vegetables, dried fruit, pickled foods, processed meats, and salad dressings)

9. Peanuts

10. Mustard

11. Wheat

12. Lupin

13. Soybeans

14. Mollusk (mussels, clams, oysters, and oyster sauce)

Chemical

Although you might strive to keep your food preparation and storage area as clean as possible, the chemicals that you use, for example, antibacterial spray or fumigation chemicals, could end up contaminating your food as well. Even before purchase, your food may also be sprayed with fertilizers and pesticides that are not good for human consumption. So, always keep all your food completely covered while cleaning the area and wash your food thoroughly before cooking or preparing.

Now that you know how to store food, this chapter will take you through where to store food, how to create your foods to create your food storage checklist, and how to preserve your own food.

But, first, there is a framework to help you remember how to manage your relationship with food during a disaster:

- **G**row your own.

- **A**lways store well.

- **P**reserve your own.

- **S**tore plenty.

WHERE TO STORE FOOD

Remember that you are storing plenty. Calories are very good in a survival situation! You never know when your food will run out, so don't take chances. Store as much as you can; use every space available to you!

Sometimes it's difficult to pinpoint places to store your food—especially if you are not a seasoned prepper. To help you along, here is a list of potential places to store your food:

Basement Storage Room

A cool, dark basement is a great place to store your food. The ideal condition for storing food is in cool, dark spaces. If your basement typically gets too hot or cold, then it is not a great place to store your food. You can build shelves in your basement to give you more space for storing your food.

Food Storage Closet

Closets in your house will often have extra space to store some food. Even just placing a box filled with cans in your clothes closet will work. You should also be able to find space in your closets to add shelves and create more space for food storage.

Over the Door Shelf Storage

This works just like a food storage closet. If there is a space over your wall, you can hang a couple of shelves to hold your food. It may not be a good idea, however, if you live in a place that's prone to earthquakes or other natural disasters.

Under the Bed Storage

You can place food in storage boxes under your bed. Simply ensure that you do not choose food in breakable containers, like glass jars, to avoid accidents.

Storage Furniture

Use furniture that comes with storage. Sofas, coffee tables and most furniture can come with adequate storage space. If you have an empty wall, then you can also place a storage cabinet there to store extra food.

Laundry Room Storage

Just like over-the-door storage, you can place shelves in strategic positions in your laundry room, for example, above your washer and dryer. Laundry rooms rarely have windows.

So, you will need to consider how to provide adequate ventilation to prevent your food from spoiling.

Under the Stairs

If you have space under your stairs, you can turn it into a storage closet. You will need to consider how to provide adequate ventilation when storing food under the stairs.

Trailers, Campers, and Boats

Trailers, stored campers, and boats will store your food well, although only for a short time. Thanks to temperature fluctuations, they do not provide ideal conditions for long-term food storage. You will need to rotate the food frequently. The one good advantage of storing food in your camper is that you can evacuate quickly in the case of an emergency.

Garage and Shed Storage

The good news is that, if you have a garage or shed, you can put up plenty of shelves to store your food. The bad news is that if your garage or shed does not have temperature control, your food will go bad very quickly thanks to temperature fluctuations. We prefer to think of garages and sheds as short-term storage solutions. Since your food will go bad quickly, it is best to use the food stored in your garage or shed first during a disaster. You will also need to rotate supplies in your garage/shed fairly regularly.

Root Cellars and Crawl Spaces

Root cellars and crawl spaces are another short-term storage solution. They have very humid air, so you will need to rotate your food regularly. Protect your food in moisture-proof plastic bags or containers

Buried Chest Freezer

Buried chest freezers and water-tight barrels are a great way to store your fruit and vegetables over the winter. They are also good for storing canned and jarred foods, as long as you use good quality, moisture-proof and rodent-proof barrels, and freezers.

Suitcases

Fill empty suitcases with food supplies and leave them in a cool, dry place.

STARTER FOOD STORAGE CHECKLIST

Here is a list of all the food that we recommend you have stored in your home for emergencies. This is just a guide. You can adapt this as you require, but this is a great starting point as this will be enough for a family to survive for months until you can find an alternative source of food.

1. 20lbs of rice

Rice is a must-have. If you want a quick source of carbs and calories, then rice is your best friend. It is versatile, so it is difficult to run out of recipes using rice. It is also very filling and nutritious.

We recommend you store a combination of white rice and brown rice. White rice is easier and faster to cook and it lasts longer when stored. Brown rice, on the other hand, has much more fiber, which keeps up your health in an emergency. It is also more filling and nutritious than white rice. Be aware, however, that brown rice will not last longer than a few months.

On the plus side, you have other options of rice, such as Basmati (brown and white), sticky rice, jasmine rice, wild rice, and more.

2. 20lbs of dried beans

Dried beans are another versatile source of food. Whether Pinto Beans, kidney beans, or any other form of beans, dried beans store for a long time, are nutritious, inexpensive, and can be used to create many recipes. They are also incredibly tasty and don't need many ingredients to taste delicious.

3. 20 cans of fruit

You need your micronutrients. Luckily, fruit contains many essential vitamins and minerals. Store pineapples, peaches, strawberries, pears, fruit cocktails, and whatever other fruits you desire. Fruits are also a great source of quick energy and a healthy form of dessert to boost your spirits in an emergency.

4. 20 cans of vegetables

Store as many vegetables as you can. That way, you get a full spectrum of micronutrients. You can store peas, corn, mixed fruit, asparagus, tomatoes, green beans, and so much more. We recommend you store an additional 20 cans of tomatoes because tomatoes are so versatile and can be used to make many dishes, including dishes made from rice and/or beans.

5. 20 cans of meat

You will need your iron and protein. Meat and fish are a great source of all three, so stock up on canned beef, spam, tuna, chicken, salmon, sausages, shrimp, etc...

A vegetarian diet is the most practical diet in emergency situations. However, there are times your body will still need meat/fish, especially since you are under the stress of surviving in a disaster scenario.

6. 4lbs oats

Oats are another versatile survival essential. They are packed with carbs and protein, so they fill you up for a long time, giving you the energy you need to survive a disaster/emergency. They are also versatile, with their ability to make many recipes, using only a few simple ingredients.

7. 5lbs salt

Your body needs salt to survive. It is imperative for many bodily functions and processes, so you must store enough salt to stay healthy.

8. 3 large jars of Peanut Butter

Peanut butter contains plenty of energy and nutritious fat for sustenance. It is also a source of protein and it lasts a long time on the shelf (one year) when unopened. It can also last for about two months when opened.

9. 5lbs powdered milk

You may not be able to find fresh milk during a disaster. In fact, fresh milk can become very rare to source during a disaster because of its brief shelf life. Powdered milk is, therefore, a great substitute. It is full of protein and fat, as well as other nutrients. to sustain you and keep you full. It is also a great addition to your foods and drinks, such as oatmeal, cereal, and coffee.

10. 5lbs coffee and/or 100 tea bags

The exact amount of coffee and tea bags you should buy depends on how much you drink. The coffee and tea bags also depend on what you like.

Stock up on what you like. The familiarity of your favorite flavored coffee or fruit tea bag will bring you a lot of comfort.

11. 10lbs of pasta

It is easy to find and stock pasta. Pasta is easy and fast to cook and very filling. Since it is so versatile to cook, you also won't get bored eating pasta.

12. 10 jars/cans of spaghetti/pasta sauce

On days when you are too tired to cook, or when you may not have enough energy, spaghetti sauce can be warmed up in 10 minutes to go with your pasta.

13. 20 cans of broth or soup

Soup works well for every meal. You don't need to add anything else. Simply warm it for a few minutes and you are set! You can also use it to add flavor to other meals such as rice and pasta dishes.

14. 2 large jars of powdered drink fortified with vitamin C (or an 8 lb bucket of ascorbic acid)

You need your vitamin C. Unfortunately, vitamin C is found in fresh fruits and vegetables. You can store juices, but they don't last very long unopened. It would take a lot of canned fruits and vegetables to get the recommended amount of vitamin C, therefore, a powdered drink fortified with vitamin C is your best substitute.

You can also store four jars of concentrated lemon juice. Not only is this a significant source of vitamin C, but it is also a good way of adding flavor to your food during a disaster.

Alternatively, you can purchase ascorbic acid. Our bodies cannot produce vitamin C, so you must get it from an outside source. Still, vitamin C is very important for preventing illnesses and keeping your immune system strong when you are at your most vulnerable (when you are highly stressed).

Ascorbic acid is the best form of vitamin C because it can last a long time without degrading. It is not sensitive to heat like vitamin supplements are and it can also be used during food preservation to minimize oxidation, browning, and discoloration of food.

15. 10lbs of pancake mix

When you are hungry and need something to fill you up for a long time, pancake mix will save the day. You can store a few tubs of margarine and bottles of honey to add as a nice topping. You can also use pancake mix to make crepes, which you can serve with some canned fruit.

16. 2 lbs of honey

Honey is great for strengthening the immune system, helping you to stave off coughs and colds. It will also boost your energy levels—just add a teaspoon to hot water or tea. Honey is a natural antibacterial so it can prevent infection in minor cuts and grazes.

Raw honey works best if you can get it, but this must not be given to infants.

17. 2 large jars of jam

Jam lasts a long time even after it is opened. It is a perfect food for when you need some sweetness and will go with your crepes, pancakes, or bread.

18. One extra large jug of cooking oil

You need oil for cooking. You also need the fat present in the oil to sustain your mind and body. Also, you need to eat fat to enable your body to break down and absorb fat-soluble vitamins and nutrients. You don't need too much oil when cooking. A dash of olive oil, coconut oil, or canola oil is enough to give you that satisfying feeling that oil provides. Plus, the oil adds flavor to your dishes.

19. Herbs, spices, and condiments

You don't want to eat the same food every day because it will get boring. Herbs, spices, and condiments are a great way to change the taste of your food, even if you are cooking the same thing. Buy those that you particularly enjoy. Buy those that go well with most dishes, such as garlic, chili, hot sauce, thyme, black pepper, paprika, oregano, rosemary, bay leaves, and salsa.

20. 2 large bags of hard candies

You want to stay healthy even in survival mode. This means that you do not want to eat too much sugar. However, you also need a good pick-me-up once in a while. Hard candies like lemon drops and butterscotch drops are a great way to find comfort occasionally.

You will notice that all the food on this list is very easy and practical to store and cook. While a beef wellington might sound good, it will require a lot of energy to preserve and prepare. Its aroma will also be too conspicuous, placing you in danger of theft in the process. Your best chance of survival is to store practical, simple food that can be easily combined into fresh meals with little cooking experience.

OTHER FOODS TO PROVIDE

You also want to store other calorie-dense foods that can last you a long time. You mustn't store any food that requires specialized tools to either prepare or preserve. They should be easy to cook, last for years, and be packed with nutrients your body needs.

Below is a good list of such foods:

1. Grains

Grains, such as rye, corn, barley, wheat, and spelt can be stored as long as they have less than 10 percent moisture. You can prepare most grains by soaking and cooking them.

Wheat can be stored for as long as 25 to 30 years. Using simple, traditional methods, you can bake bread using just wheat, salt, and water. You can also create your own wood fire oven as will be discussed in the next chapter. There are different varieties of wheat available to you, including gluten-free options such as einkorn.

Plan to store about 300lbs-400lbs of grain per person. If you can purchase a small grain mill, do so. It enables you to grind wheat and grains to use to make tortillas and bread. It also makes your home look like a traditional farmstead, which is a great additional benefit.

2. Potato flakes

Potato flakes are quick to prepare in just a few minutes. All you need is boiling water. They are also a great way to thicken your stews and soups and make them more calorie-dense.

Even better, they contain a high number of micronutrients that your body needs to survive.

3. Dehydrated and Freeze-Dried vegetables

It is a no-brainer why you need dehydrated and freeze-dried vegetables. They are packed with nutrients and fiber and they add taste to your food. Onions, carrots, and celery are the most important dried vegetables you need. Onions and celery, in particular, add a lot of flavor to your food, while carrots are a rare source of vitamin A for preppers.

4. White sugar

As we've already discussed, you don't want to eat too much sugar as a survivalist. It is not only bad for your overall health but your oral health as well during a time when you may not find a dentist. Nonetheless, sugar is a great preservative. In the next part of this chapter, we will talk about the different ways to preserve food, one of which is sugar. Store about 70lbs of sugar per person.

5. Baking Soda

Baking soda is a wonderfully versatile food product. You can use it for cooking, baking, cleaning, personal hygiene, and medicinal uses. This cheap powder with an infinite shelf-life is a must-have for your survival kitchen. Store 10lbs of baking soda per person.

6. Vinegar

Like baking soda, vinegar has a lot of uses for both cooking and non-cooking. It is used in many recipes and for preserving food by pickling and acidifying. It has great medicinal uses, such as relieving indigestion, and is a brilliant disinfectant and cleaner.

There are a variety of kinds of vinegar available to you, so we recommend you store them according to their primary use: white distilled vinegar is great for cleaning and bottling; rice vinegar is perfect for creating delicious dishes, and apple cider vinegar has wonderful medicinal and cleaning properties. Store 4 gallons of vinegar for cleaning and 2 gallons of vinegar per person for cooking, preserving, and medicinal uses.

PRESERVING YOUR OWN

Now that you've learned how to store well, it is time to learn how to preserve well. Storing food for a family of 4 to last for months can be very expensive. One way to reduce your expenses is to grow your own food and preserve it. In fact, learning how to preserve your food is a lifelong skill that will serve you well, no matter your situation.

It is a great way to stop relying on archaic government-assisted food distribution systems and corporate supermarkets and learn to lean on yourself instead. We like to think that, although we can't trust many people or corporations in life, we can trust ourselves.

Therefore, the more skills you learn for survival, the more you can trust yourself no matter what situation you find yourself in. The skill of preserving your food is easy. You can preserve food by:

1. Canning

Almost any food can be canned, from fruits to vegetables to soups. To can your food, you will need to invest in a home canning kit. It will contain the following equipment:

- 1 pressure canner

- Quart or pint cans

- Can lids and bands (both wide mouth and regular)*

- Can lifter

- Canning rack (optional equipment to use when water bath canning)

- Can Funnel

- Canning salt

Note: Always use new lids. Never reuse lids when canning to avoid contamination.

The kit will cost you about $200. If you plan on canning just fruit, a water bath canner is good enough because the high acidity of the fruit will kill all bacteria.

To can your fresh produce at home, ensure the fruits are juicy and ripe and the vegetables are crisp. Wash them thoroughly, then cut off the blooms. Blanch the vegetables, killing all bacteria, and then can.

Ensure cooked food, such as meat, chili, and soup, is cooked thoroughly before canning.

2. Dehydrating

Moisture gives bacteria the ideal environment for growth. By dehydrating your food, you prevent bacteria from growing, causing your food to last a long time. Dehydration has been used for centuries, especially in hot countries where food spoils quickly. Today, thanks to electric dehydrators, dehydrating your food is very safe. You can dehydrate meat, fish, spices, fruit, and vegetables. Once dehydrated, food can last for years.

Even better, there are delicious recipes online for dehydrating your food. This way you don't have to have the same old dehydrated fruit or vegetables. You can mix it up to have a delicious variety of dehydrated food on hand for survival. These dehydrators typically cost between $60 and $250, depending on the quality you want.

Dehydrating food involves washing it and then drying it thoroughly. It is a skill that requires a fair bit of practice, especially since fresh foods need different methods of dehydration. We recommend cookbooks or video tutorials to help you get started.

3. Smoking

To smoke meat, you essentially dry it over wood chips to give it an additional layer of flavor. Using different types of wood chips will give you a distinct flavor to your meat. For example, beef jerky is made from smoked meat.

4. Root cellar

A root cellar is like nature's pantry. It keeps your food at a stable temperature, with the right amount of humidity to keep it fresh for long. You will need to make sure that you use wood shelving because wood shelving retains neither cold nor heat. It also allows for good air circulation, which food needs to stay fresh.

Likewise, food stored in root cellars needs to be kept with plenty of space in between to allow for air circulation. These fresh produce store well in root cellars:

- Carrots

- Onions

- Pumpkins

- Cabbage

- Potatoes

- Squash

- Pears

- Beets

- Turnips

- Apples

- Leeks

- Garlic

- Unripened tomatoes

To store your produce in a root cellar, harvest them without washing off the soil. The soil will keep the produce cool, preserving them. Lay them flat on the shelves and check that none of them are bruised. Bruised and rotten produce stored with healthy produce will rot the whole batch of produce with alarming speed. You can lose all your produce just from one bruised or rotten crop, so be very careful to check for these before storing them.

5. Curing

Curing uses the same processes as smoking and dehydration. When curing food, you take out all the moisture from the food using sea salt or kosher salt, preventing bacteria from growing as a result. After salting the meat, you have to hang it up to dry, ensuring that air can reach it from both sides to draw out all the moisture evenly.

6. Sugaring

Sugaring is like curing. A surface coated with crystal or granulated sugar is inhospitable to bacteria. To sugar a food, dry it completely first, then coat the surface in sugar. While sugared meats and vegetables may not taste nice, they are still foods that will ensure your survival. Sugared fruit is, of course, delicious.

7. Pickling

When you pickle food, you place it in antimicrobial conditions that are severely inhospitable for bacteria. This usually means placing it in brine or vinegar. You can pickle very many foods, including meats, eggs, vegetables, and even some fruits. Like sugaring, pickling food can change the texture and taste of the food. However, when in survival mode, you are more concerned with getting enough calories and nutrients than the taste or texture of your food. Luckily, your brain is so focused on achieving this goal in survival mode that you can wolf down food that you would turn your nose up at in everyday life.

8. Fermentation

Fermenting foods involves breaking down the carbohydrates in food and converting them into alcohol or acids to preserve them. Fermentation is the process we use to create cheese, beer, and yogurt. It is one of the oldest methods for preserving food in human history, so you will find plenty of tutorials and instructions on how to ferment your food.

GROWING YOUR OWN

To preserve your own food, you have to first grow your own food. Growing your own food is a skill that will benefit you in most situations in life. Unfortunately, most people today have become too complacent, comfortable, and lazy to grow their food. Thanks to their over-reliance on supermarkets and takeout restaurants, you will have noticed that people are becoming not only lazy but obese and unhealthy.

For people like you who want to stay healthy and live long, growing your food is a great way to avoid the poison and the complacency of modern living. It is a wonderful reversion to the traditional way of life that served our grandparents very well.

When you grow your own food, you eat a healthier, more nutritious diet. What's more, you are more active because you are always in your garden, working the land. Indeed, there are a lot of ways in which growing your own food benefits you as a prepper—ways that will be discussed in more depth in Chapter 11.

SURVIVAL TASK

Answer the following questions:

- How much food do you currently have stored?

- Do you have a rough food plan?

293

- How long will this last you?

- Do you feel that, if you were faced with a disaster scenario, you could feed yourself comfortably?

Check in with these questions, making sure you have a plan, or that you are, at least, thinking about making a plan. This is vital to be fully prepared for a variety of likely outcomes. One such outcome is a lack of power during a disaster. Without electricity, our traditional methods of preserving food become useless. So, alternative methods for preservation are really important. Likewise, without electricity, our traditional methods of cooking food also become useless, as will be examined in the next chapter.

Key Chapter Takeaway

- You can store all the food in the world, but if you come back to your food during a disaster to find that it has been contaminated, then all your hard work would have amounted to nothing.

- There are four types of contamination that come from not properly storing food: microbial, physical, allergenic, and chemical.

- Ideally, you want to store your food in a cool and dry basement storage room or pantry, placed on sturdy shelves that allow you to access and rotate your food regularly.

- Ideally, you also just want to start with what you have and slowly build on that.

- Ensure that your food is always stored on heavy-duty shelving to prevent spills and breakage and rotate your food regularly to avoid eating expired food.

- When storing food, store food that is very easy and practical to store and cook.

- Store calorie-dense foods that can last you a long time.

- Storing food for a family of 4 to last for months can be very expensive. One way to reduce your expenses is to grow your own food and preserve it.

- For people who want to stay healthy and live long, growing your own food is a great way to avoid the poison and the complacency and poison of modern living.

In the next chapter, you will learn how to cook your food with no electricity or power.

CHAPTER FIVE:
SURVIVAL COOKERY

In a disaster situation, conventional cooking techniques may be useless since they often rely on piped gas or electricity, which might not be available. Therefore, it is important to have other options.

This chapter will teach you how to cook food without power and how to create an outdoor oven to cook the food you stored. Now you know how to store enough food, you need to know how to cook it too. Although much of the food you store can be eaten cold, having a hot meal can do so much for your morale. Plus, you will still need to cook your carbs, grains, and legumes.

Survival cooking, at its heart, is creative cooking. You need to think of alternative ways to cook your food without an electric cooker, oven, or microwave on hand. Using the framework: O.U.T., you can keep in mind the different options available to you for cooking.

- **O**ven cooking

- **U**nconventional cooking.

- **T**raditional cooking.

WAYS TO COOK FOOD WITHOUT POWER

One of the most bizarre parts of experiencing a disaster is the lack of energy. We are so used to energy that we take it for granted. But once it is gone, you realize just how much we rely on and depend on energy for survival. For one, many foods need to be cooked to become ingestible and digestible. Even if you eat them raw, your body cannot break them down small enough to extract the much-needed vitamins and minerals. For another, many perishable foods go bad surprisingly fast if not placed in the fridge or freezer.

Familiarizing yourself with ways to cook food without power is a much-needed survival skill that will keep you fed, healthy and happy during a disaster.

Some of the best ways of cooking food without power are the more traditional methods. These are methods we often use when camping, hiking, or simply going outdoors. They continue to be popular despite the advancements in electrical cooking methods because they are tried and tested methods of cooking a nice, hot, tasty meal when electricity is not practical. As well as the traditional methods of cooking outdoors, this chapter will include some more unconventional methods that you may never have heard of before, methods that will be incredibly useful when you are starving and need to eat.

Without power, you can cook using:

1. BBQ grill

A backyard barbeque grill or smoker is a handy way to cook your food. It is most likely that you have used one before or you have seen others use it before, so it doesn't take too long to master. Also, you can choose to use a dual propane/charcoal BBQ grill. With a dual grill, you can choose to use one source of fuel if you run out of the other. It is also helpful because you can pick up sticks and pieces of wood to burn for fuel should you run out of both charcoal and propane.

Another advantage is that you can cook side dishes or boil water using a barbecue grill that comes with a side burner.

As always, store plenty of charcoal (and wood), as well as tanks full of propane to last you months without power.

Barbecue grills can be quite big and heavy, especially if you need to cook for a large survival party. Consequently, you will need to consider where to store your barbecue grill.

2. Open fire

Most people have experience cooking on an open fire. Whether it's roasting chestnuts, marshmallows, roasting meat, or warming up a can of beans while camping, an open fire has always been an ever-present source of cooking for mankind. All you will need is clean burning wood and a fire-safe, non-toxic metal stands to place your cooking pans and kettles over the open fire. It takes a bit of practice to start one and to use one effectively, but a few tries are enough to give you the experience you need.

Be careful when using open fires to avoid the fire spreading and destroying the surrounding area.

3. Volcano stoves

A volcano stove is a small, portable stove, often used for camping purposes. They are collapsible and easy to store, taking up very little space, unlike BBQ grills. Even better, they are just as efficient whether fueled by propane, charcoal, or wood. They can be stored as an alternative to a barbecue grill in case of emergencies.

4. Solar ovens

Solar ovens are a great alternative to conventional cooking if you will be bugging in within your own home. The best advantage of a solar oven is that it requires no energy source since it is powered by the sun. Nonetheless, it is not a good primary source of cooking because you cannot cook during overcast days. You will also be limited to cooking between 11:00 am and 4:00 pm on sunny days.

Solar ovens trap the heat of the sun using a solar panel. This heat is transferred to the stove, which then cooks your food. A solar oven does not differ significantly from leaving your can of soup in the sun to heat. The only difference is you trap the heat to heat or cook your food faster in a solar oven.

Some solar ovens do not work well, so do your research before making a purchase. Sometimes, the paint inside solar ovens peels off. You should keep high-temperature barbecue black spray paint on hand to respray it when this happens.

5. Camp stoves

Propane camp stoves are a handy non-conventional cooking method. They need to be fueled by propane and must be used outdoors. Camp stoves are also usually small, so you won't be able to cook much food on it at the same time.

6. Fondue sets

Fondue sets are magnificent for heating food during a disaster—as long as you use an alcohol-burning one. It also means you will need to store some cooking alcohol on hand along with your other alternative sources of power.

UNCONVENTIONAL COOKING   TECHNIQUES

There are a lot of ways for cooking and heating your food. You just need to be creative. Your primary goal when cooking or heating food is to get it hot. What we mean by this is that you need a source of heat. Once you find a source of heat, the rest is history.

Likewise, as a prepper, you must have an emergency plan for your emergencies. It may sound silly but, simply put, when you are in a disaster and you don't have your traditional cooking methods on hand, you need another emergency cooking method to cover your original disaster cooking plan. A good prepper always has a Plan B, should your Plan A not work out. A great prepper will also have a back-up Plan C, should Plan B fail.

Unconventional cooking methods are your Plan B for your traditional cooking methods. Some good unconventional cooking methods for emergencies include:

1. Canned heat

Canned heat is also known as Sterno or gelled fuel. It is made from alcohol, which is then turned into a burnable jelly. You can purchase canned heat online from shopping retailers. You can also search camping stores and retailers that stock survival gear. Always keep a few supplies of canned heat in case of emergencies.

Be aware, however, that Canned Heat can be hard to contain just like an alcohol stove; and that the flame of canned heat can be hard to contain, just like an alcohol stove. They are also quite expensive to purchase, so you cannot stock too much of it. This is okay since you are only stocking a few supplies for emergencies only.

On the plus side, since they are made of alcohol jelly, canned heat doesn't evaporate and will, therefore, last, even when stored over a long period.

2. Tuna can and toilet paper stove

The tuna can and toilet paper stove is used by specialized armed forces internationally. Not only is it a great source of heat but it also makes a good emergency light.

Here is how to build one:

1. Open a small to medium can of tuna in oil, or any other can that has been used to store oil, like a can of sardines in oil.

2. Place 3 pieces of toilet paper flat over the tuna pieces so that they absorb the oil.

3. Once the toilet paper absorbs the oil, the toilet paper will create an airtight seal around the lid of the tuna can.

4. Light the toilet paper with a source of fire. The stove should burn for about 25 minutes–enough time to cook some food.

5. The fire will also cook the tuna underneath the toilet paper, which you can also then eat afterward.

3. Buddy burner

A buddy burner is quite similar to a tuna can stove except, this time, you empty the tuna can first.

Here is how to build one:

1. Cut out cardboard strips that are slightly thinner than the height of your tuna can. Ensure that you cut across the corrugated part. This way, the holes will be exposed on the sides.

2. Place them inside your empty tuna can.

3. Roll the strips of cardboard tightly, then fit them snugly inside the tuna can.

4. Melt either crayon or candle wax in a separate tin or pan, then pour onto the strips of cardboard. Never melt wax over a direct flame because it will easily catch fire.

5. Pour the melted wax over the cardboard strips. You can also use melted butter in place of melted wax.

6. Fill all the holes in the cardboard, and leave a bit of the cardboard roll exposed. This exposed cardboard will serve as the wick. Alternatively, stick a small piece of cardboard inside the can to use as a lighting wick. This will make it slightly easier to light your buddy burner.

7. Leave the wax to harden, then light your buddy burner. Once the wax hardens, you can light the buddy burner. You can stick a small piece of cardboard inside to serve as a wick and make lighting it easier if you wish.

4. Hay box oven

A hay box oven is as its name suggests. It is a box oven that traps heat. Once you heat your pot of food, for example, outside on an outdoor fire, you place it in the hay box oven. You then place hay all around the pot, close the box and leave it for 8-12 hours for the food to be cooked.

Hay box ovens work by trapping thermal heat and using this trapped heat to complete the cooking process. It is a great way to cook food that needs to be simmered over low heat for a long time, such as legumes and stews. Think of it as an emergency slow cooker. It works great if you can't stayoutside for 12 hours, constantly checking up on your food, for example, if it is too cold or too hot outside. It is also great because you need very little fuel using a hay box oven since it relies on its own trapped heat.

Another significant benefit is that you can make your hay box oven should you need to do so. All you will need is an insulated box, for example, a cooler that you no longer use. You will then also need something insulated to place on top and beside your cooler to trap the thermal heat in, for instance, a cardboard box that you line with aluminum foil, as well as old, thick sweaters and blankets.

5. Tea light oven

Tea light ovens, also known as Home Emergency Radiant Cooking (HERC), work using tea lights. It works by using multiple tea lights at once to cook over a small pot. This is only an emergency use of tea lights because it will take up to 8 hours to cook a small pot of food. You will need to use an enclosed pot and place it atop of the tea lights. By doing so, the pot will trap heat and simmer the food.

As with the hay box oven, a tea light oven can be used for slow cooking over low heat. You can cook food like stews, soups, and mac and cheese over a tea light oven.

Remember that these techniques are more for emergency-based cooking. A more long-term method would be more appropriate (as discussed in the next part of this chapter). However, for emergencies, these would work well.

CREATING A WOOD-FIRED EARTH OVEN

Whether you are bugging in your own home or bugging out elsewhere (as will be discussed in the next chapter), creating a wood-fired earth oven is a long-term solution for ensuring that you have a cooking method that does not rely on conventional cooking techniques.

Wood-fired ovens have been used for centuries by civilizations all over the world. Most societies have had a version of their wood-fired oven specifically because it works very well and is highly reliable. We see a wood-fired earth oven as a permanent replacement for an electric cooker or electric oven.

Even better, with a wood-fired earth oven, you do not have to rely on unconventional or traditional cooking methods unless in emergencies, or unless you only want to cook a little food and don't fancy lighting a whole fire in the oven.

If you live in a cold climate, a wood-fired earth oven is another way to keep warm when it is cold. Some societies traditionally built their ovens inside their homes as a source of heat and fire. We wouldn't recommend you build your oven indoors because modern homes have too many flammable materials.

BENEFITS OF A WOOD-FIRED OVEN

There are other great benefits of building your wood-fired oven. They include:

305

- You can bake a lot of delicious foods, including soft bread, crusty bread, and pizzas.

- It works like an electric oven. You can roast meats and fish, as well as baked dishes, such as savory and sweet pies and even cakes.

- It is very cheap to make since your key ingredient is the clay on the ground.

BUILD YOUR OWN WOOD-FIRED OVEN

Here is a detailed step-by-step guide for creating a wood-fired earth oven:

1. **The first steps for making your wood-fired earth oven**

Ensure you have enough mud to make the oven. The amount of clay you need depends on the size of the oven you want to build. While you can't gauge exactly how much clay you need, if you have enough clay covering the ground of your property, then this should be sufficient.

Get together all the tools you need, mainly a wheelbarrow, a shovel, a tape measure, some large buckets, scraps of wood, a plastic tarp, red bricks, and sculpting tools (kitchen utensils will work well for this).

Your next step is to prepare a base for the oven. You can prepare the base on the ground. Conversely, if you plan to use your oven frequently, then place your base at a waist-length level. You do not want to have to bend to the ground every time you need to put in or take out your food from the oven.

If you decide to place your oven base at waist-length, raise the base using miscellaneous objects, such as broken-up concrete, logs, or rocks.

2. Making the wood-fired oven floor

Your next step is to make the oven floor. A good measurement is between 20 and 27 inches. If you plan to bake things that are taller than 27 inches, then make the floor larger.

Lay red or fire bricks on prepared tamped sand that has been smoothed. The sand must be between 4 to 6 inches deep. You can also use used mortar-free bricks.

To set the bricks. set one brick leveled and solid. Next, hold the second brick level, just above the sand, gently setting its long side to the long side of the first brick. Continue this process, setting each brick down flat and firm without wiggling them. Tap down bricks so that they are all level with each other.

3. Making a form

Pile moist sand on the set bricks, then shape them to a few inches higher than half of the oven floor's width. For example, if your oven is 24 inches wide, the sand form should be 12 inches high.

Calculate the interior height by measuring the distance from the top to the floor. Multiply this height by 63% to determine the measurement for your oven door.

4. Mixing mud for your outdoor oven

You must use soil below the topsoil to build your oven. You can either mix one part clay with one to three parts sharp (builder's) sand or use it as it is. Note that pure clay subsoil usually shrinks and cracks more than a sand mix. You can find soil in your backyard, road cuts, construction sites, or river banks.

To verify that it is clay subsoil, check that it feels slippery, sticky, and a bit greasy (not crumbly and floury). Wet the soil by adding water a little at a time. Use your hands and feet to mix, but check for debris first. You can also just use your feet by stomping with boots on. Mix until it begins to clump like pie crust dough, or until you can roll the dough into snakelike ropes that bend easily. To test it, drop a ball from chest height. If it breaks, add a little water.

Make a test brick. Once dried, the brick would be hard and dense with little to no cracks.

5. Build your wood-fired oven

Lay sheets of wet newspaper flat on your sand form. This stops the mud walls from sticking to the sand form. Cover the sand form with a 3-4 inches thick layer of mud, maintaining an even thickness. You will cut out the doorway later, so don't worry about that.

Once the oven dome form is completed, pack the mud material using a flat board until it sits solidly against the form. It shouldn't stick to the board but, if it does, your mix is too damp and needs to dry for longer. Once you confirm the first layer is dried, add more layers. Last, add a fine finish plaster, if you so desire.

6. Remove the oven sand dome form

Your doorway needs to be 63 percent of the height of your oven. Its width should be 33-50 percent of the oven's inner diameter. Outline in the mud where you want the door to be, then slowly carve out the door, stopping once you hit the newspaper layer. But first, press gently on the outline with your fingers. If it leaves a dent, it is not dry enough to be dug out. Wait until it feels like leather, then try again. Be patient as this step can take days, and even weeks!

7. Make your outdoor oven beautiful

Polish the outside of your oven. You can draw patterns on the surface or build a mud extension, like a bench. You should also think about building a roof with sticks and mud.

No matter how you choose to decorate, do not cover the oven with cement or paint. It needs to breathe, otherwise, trapped moisture will render it useless.

8. Making the oven door

Finally, cut out the door. It doesn't need to be a perfect fit as wet cloth draped over it adds much-needed moisture to your food when baking. Your oven is now ready to use, barring one step.

Build your first fire and allow the smoke to come out. There will be no more black soot on the inside of the dome once the oven is dry (after two-three hours). Your oven is now ready to use.

By preparing this oven in advance, you will be ready to go off-grid, whether or not there is a catastrophe. There are other benefits, such as making great pizza nights! Even if you have never experienced a disaster or emergency, having a wood-fired oven still has many great uses. Since they last for many decades, if built well, you are guaranteed to use them for your entire life. In that case, they are a substantial investment no matter how you look at it.

SURVIVAL TASK

Try a few of the emergency cooking methods after finishing the chapter. This means you will know exactly what to do should the worst happen and you'll be prepared for the worst.

Key Chapter Takeaway

- Survival cooking is, at its heart, creative cooking.

- You need to think of alternative ways to cook your food without an electric cooker, oven, or microwave on hand or you will starve.

- Many foods need to be cooked to become ingestible and digestible. If you try to eat them raw, your body cannot extract the much-needed vitamins and minerals.

- Some of the best ways of cooking food without power are the more traditional, tried, and true methods. These are methods we often use when camping, hiking, or simply outdoors.

- The most important thing when cooking food without power is to find a source of heat.

- When you are in a disaster and you don't have your traditional cooking methods on hand, you need another emergency cooking method to cover your original disaster cooking plan.

- Most societies have a version of their wood-fired oven because it works very well and is highly reliable.

- A wood-fired earth oven is a permanent replacement for an electric cooker or electric oven.

- By preparing this oven in advance, you will be prepared for going off grid, whether or not there is a catastrophe.

In the next chapter, you will learn how to create shelters in case you need to evacuate your home.

CHAPTER SIX:
CREATING SHELTER

Although you will prefer to bug-in at home during an emergency, in situations where you would have to evacuate your home, it is essential to have other shelters or safe houses prepared. As we said in the previous chapter, a good prepper always has a Plan B to cover Plan A, should your Plan A not work out. A great prepper will also have a back-up Plan C, should Plan B fail.

The rule of 3 states that you need three things to survive: air, water, and food. These are your three foremost concerns after a disaster. Once you've taken care of these needs, you will want to focus on another basic necessity for survival: shelter.

Have you ever stopped to consider why humans of all civilizations and cultures have built some sort of shelter, even if it might just be a makeshift tent? Well, because sleeping outside in the rain for hours is not ideal. Neither is sitting in the sun during a heat wave, being exposed not just to the elements, but to predators and venomous creatures and critters. Consequently, in the hierarchy of human survival, shelter comes after the rule of 3.

In fact, most times, shelter can be more important than water and food. Why? Well, you can die within the space of a few hours in unideal conditions. Essentially, it is impossible for you to go out looking for water if you cannot find shelter to protect yourself from a storm for a few hours.

Shelter protects you from long-term exposure to the elements and the outside world, which could cause hypothermia (becoming too cold), hyperthermia (becoming too hot), and many other dangerous conditions. Your body is always trying to thermoregulate itself. This means that it is always trying to keep you at a constant human temperature of 98.6°F (37°C) in order to keep you alive.

Shelter is simply your way of empowering your body to do its job of keeping you alive and well. The only thing that will kill you faster than a lack of shelter is a lack of air. We like to think of it this way: you can survive a day in a good, dry, warm shelter without water. However, you can be as hydrated and satiated as you want, but you will not survive a day out in the snow without shelter.

Humans have many more ways of keeping warm without shelter, such as coats, fur, and fire, but these are only temporary measures. You will need shelter after only a few days.

Ideally, a shelter should be able to not just keep you at the human temperature, but even warmer. It should keep you dry, repelling wind and rain, and be able to radiate heat off of human bodies to keep the entire shelter warm. Additionally, it should be able to conserve heat from other sources, like fire, and give you the ability to sleep off the ground, so that you do not lose your body heat. Last, it should be able to provide shade, but also keep you cool in hot temperatures.

When we talk about shelter, most people think of big comfortable tents or even cabins. The good news is you don't have to build a cabin unless you want to. Something as simple as a tent made of sticks and a reflective blanket, or a cave tunneled out of a snowbank, will meet all these conditions.

Thankfully today, we also have many more sophisticated ways of building makeshift shelters, whether long-term or short-term. This chapter will explore the options available to you, including bug-out shelters, bunkers, and other longer-term shelters. But, first, you must remember to be **PIOUS** when thinking of shelter. That means that:

- **P**repare to bug in and out.

- **I**n a disaster, everyone is an enemy.

- **O**n the move, build temporary shelters.

- **U**nderground bunkers are Plan C.

- **S**helter before food and water.

BUGGING IN VS BUGGING OUT

Before we get into the different options available to you, however, you need to understand the key pros and cons of bugging out and bugging in. These are very common terms thrown around in the prepper community, so you might wonder how to choose which is the best option for you in different disaster scenarios. This table will help you figure out the benefits and downsides to both bugging in and bugging out.

	Bugging In	Bugging Out
PROS	If someone in your survival party is physically unable to travel long distances or has medical needs, bugging in is the clear winner.	When shit hits the fan, bugging out can keep you from deadly disease or violence, you can avoid becoming infected or hurt by going off-grid.
	Bugging in is much less stressful than bugging out. You don't have to carry heavy things, worry about leaving something essential behind,	Preparing to bug-out removes the anxiety of a possible disaster. You are more flexible because you are ready to leave at any time.

	or about making shelter.	
	Houses are very reliable and keep us safe from the elements - very cold, winter conditions and very hot summer conditions.	You have more space when you bug-out for gardening, hunting, and other survival techniques.
	You get the familiarity of being around people who know you. Your neighbor is much more likely to look out for you and share with you, and vice versa. By building a survival	You have to learn a lot of skills to be able to bug out. While it is a lot of work, these skills will never leave you.

	community, you are more likely to survive.	
	You have a well-stocked survival pantry, meaning you don't have to forage or hunt for food. You also have more places to hide your food, in case of break-ins.	You don't have to worry about being hit by either natural or artificial disasters. You can choose to bug-out in a location that is free of both human interference and a history of natural disasters.
CONS	You could be caught in civil unrest, riots, and other deadly, violent eruptions in urban and suburban areas.	Bugging out is stressful for the elderly, sick, children, and pets, so use it only as a final option if you have any of these in your survival party.

	In an area that regularly has natural disasters, bugging in can have severe risks. It may be the least safe choice.	You are only able to carry limited medical supplies. Any disease, accident, or illness could be hard to treat, even an emergency phone call might be too late by the time emergency services get to you.
	Your neighbors, even if they know you very well, can turn against you. Remember that disaster brings out the worst in humans. If you have supplies, you have to be prepared to defend yourself.	You can only carry enough food for a few days before you need to start looking for your food, either by hunting or foraging.

	The COVID-19 pandemic showed us that governments can– and will–keep citizens from leaving their homes or even moving freely. If you decide to bug in, you could become trapped, with no supplies, and when disaster worsens.	Bugging out requires a lot of physical exertion. You will get very tired and depleted of essential nutrients and electrolytes. You need to be physically fit to survive bugging out.
	Bugging in will mean that you have limited space. Your family may start to feel suffocated the longer you have to stay in this one space to survive.	You will need to defend yourself against possible predators, harmful animals, looters, or any other person who may want to harm you.

Based on the pros and cons in the table above, it might be tempting to think that one method is better than another.

You will want to choose either bugging out or bugging in because one method will suit your specific situation better.

Nevertheless, we would advise you not to be tempted to think that just one option will work for you. Remember, always have a Plan A, a Plan B, and a Plan C. In this case, you can only have two plans, so choose both.

This means that you choose one primary method of survival, but also prepare for the second method as a backup option. The method you choose will be whichever one applies best to you, has less risk, and has a higher chance of survival, based on the pros and cons. So, while you may prepare your house with two years' worth of food supply for bugging in, you will also need to learn how to defend yourself as a contingency plan, should you need to leave your home and bug out.

Ways To Fortify Your Home To Bug In

As you've seen from the table above, one con of bugging-in is that you may have to deal with looters or even violent rioters. In a disaster, everyone is an enemy. What this really means is that anyone can turn on you once the desperation for food, water, air, shelter, or medicine gets to them. So, the best way to defend yourself is to fortify your home. This reduces your need to use force and violence.

To fortify your home for bugging in:

1. Never spill the beans.

A good prepper is secretive. That means you never tell people you are a prepper.

Other than the people in your survival party, nobody else must know that you keep drinkable water and a year's food supply because once shit hits the fan, they will come knocking. If you refuse to help them, things will quickly turn violent against you and your survival party.

There are other ways for people to find out that you are a prepper without you speaking about it. For example, they could find receipts from your purchases, or they could smell your cooking or see you drinking a glass of juice when the juice has not been sold in supermarkets for months.

Hence, you need to camouflage yourself so that, from the outside, you look to be living the same life like everyone else around you during a disaster. Tear up receipts after purchase. Dress the same and act the same. Cover your windows and lock all windows and doors when cooking. You may even think about complaining to your neighbors about not having enough to eat. Yes, it is manipulative, but once the shit hits the fan, the societal rules change and it is a survival of the fittest situation. It is better to be manipulative than end up dead because a hungry neighbor looted your home for food.

2. Defend your perimeter.

The best offense is a good defense, so guard your perimeter. It is best to simply keep people from entering your home in the first place. However, you need to be inconspicuous about it. If you suddenly put up a tall fence, your neighbors will realize that you have something to protect. Defend your perimeter by putting barbed wire and broken glass on the fence and on the surrounding perimeter near the fence.

Plant defensive plants that are very thorny and have loads of prickles, like the century plant, firethorn, tomato porcupine, bougainvillea, and Spanish bayonet. They are nature's barbed wire.

You can also use trees and shrubs to stop others from looking into your home. However, do so strategically, so that you also can see if anyone else is looking into your home, trying to snoop and find ways of breaking in.

Ensure that there is open space between the fence and your actual home so that you can see whoever is outside trying to get in. Don't be afraid to use warning signs, such as "trespassers will be shot." Although, if you do have a dog on the premises, do not use a warning sign advertising this as your pet could be stolen for food.

Last, good old-fashioned hidden cameras and motion lights work superbly well. Use a solar-charged one in case of power outages.

3. Fortify your home.

The next step of protection from anyone who makes it past your perimeter is the outer area of your home, including your walls, doors, and windows. Use heavy, solid wood or metal-insulated doors and install them with longer set screws and strike plates. Add high-quality, single-cylinder deadbolt locks and door jammers.

Door jammers could save your life by buying you some time to escape. Secure your window sills with defensive plants and install burglar bars over your windows. Install window locks and add security film to your window panes to strengthen them against breakage. Last, you can set up sandbags to defend yourself against any armed intruders using a gun.

You also have the option of setting booby traps, such as trip wires, perimeter alarms, corn flour explosives, and pit traps. Still, we don't recommend this option. They may look cool in movies, but they are deadly and can land you in legal trouble.

4. Build a safe room.

Your last option for protection in a bug-in scenario is a safe room/bunker. Stockpile your safe room or bunker with enough food and supplies to keep you alive for months. Remember to be inconspicuous. This means that your safe room does not look like any other room out of the ordinary. That way, you do not alert intruders to the purpose of this room or to the fact that you're in there.

Make sure you have enough sleeping space and moving room for every member of the survival party. You will also need to make sure it is in a location in your home where everyone in your survival party can reach quickly in case of danger or intruders.

It is difficult to find space for a safe house if your house is small. Here, you'll need to be creative to find a space that will work for you.

Bug-out Shelters

Here are some bug-out shelters that are available to you, whether you live in an urban or rural area. Be aware that these are temporary shelters that you can use for only a few weeks before you will need to find more permanent shelter. Many of these temporary shelters can be used while you are on the move to safety. Either way, they can help you wait out the disaster and its aftermath until you can safely return home.

1. Urban Bug-out Shelters

Underneath Staircases

Assuming your staircase is small, it can provide a cozy nook for waiting out a disaster, staying safe, and also hiding in case you need to.

It can be a good option, as it is structured similar to a lean-to and one can tuck in behind and be fairly invisible. You will feel cramped/claustrophobic if you have to stay there for more than a few weeks.

Shipping Containers

Shipping containers are ready-made, sturdy, totally weatherproof, and you can find them all over the place. They will block out wind and water—if they are in good shape—and keep you safe from dangerous animals.

If you choose one that looks dilapidated on the outside and is in a remote area, you will also be safe from other people. If someone stumbles across one, they might wander in, looking for shelter and/or supplies too. You will also need to be very careful not to accidentally lock yourself in.

Dumpster Shelters

The first thing you think of when you hear dumpsters is the horrible smell. Yet, dumpsters are a great temporary shelter if you can withstand the smell or find one that doesn't smell too bad. As with shipping containers, dumpsters attract both people and animals looking for food, shelter, and other supplies. They do protect you from the rain and wind and they are found almost everywhere.

To prevent unwanted visitors, wrap cordage around the lid, then tie it around your waist.

2. Rural Bug-out Shelters

Lean-To Shelters

A lean-to is the easiest temporary shelter to construct. You only need some building scraps and a couple of large pieces of cardboard to build one.

You can also search for insulating materials, like styrofoam, to keep you off the ground so you can stay warm and dry. Alternatively, you can use wooden pallets to stay off the ground.

As with most temporary shelters, one of your main concerns is staying hidden. People searching for supplies will target your lean-to. Hide your shelter behind debris or any leftover scrap once you complete your lean-to.

Debris Hut

We like to think of debris huts as nature's sleeping bags. They naturally trap your body heat so that you can keep warm through the night. You can also build them with enough room to move around a bit so that you are not cramped.

To build your own debris hut, create a bipod with two poles, measuring four feet in length. Lay a ridge pole, measuring eight feet, against it. Lean branches on both sides, ensuring it is at a 45-degree angle. Lastly, pile several feet of debris at the top to create a thick layer of insulation.

The good thing about debris huts is that they are naturally hidden thanks to all the debris you pile on them, so most people would not even notice it. Try not to sleep on the ground. Instead, use wood pallets or insulating materials, like styrofoam.

Emergency Blanket Shelter

Emergency blankets are big enough to build a temporary shelter in most situations. Thanks to their reflective surface, however, they are very shiny, which means they will attract nearby animals and people.

You can set up an emergency blanket like you would a tarp, using any nearby sticks to keep it upright. You can also tie it to a tree or peg it down into the ground.

CREATING A BUNKER

Our mantra is that a prepper always has a Plan A and a Plan B. A good prepper also has a Plan C. Bugging in and bugging out are your Plans A and B. whichever one fits your needs will obviously be your chosen Plan A. But you should know that there is a Plan C in this case: an underground bunker. A Plan C is always nice for your peace of mind, and if you decide to go down this route, it will become Plan A. But it is still optional and if, after reading this chapter, you decide that a bunker is too expensive, or it takes too much effort, then you can skip this step in your prepping plan.

Gone are the days when people built bunkers because they were terrified of a Nuclear War. Now we are terrified of even more things that could happen, such as:

1. Natural disasters

Tornadoes

Scarily enough, natural disasters are becoming more constant. In the event of something like a tornado, you may not be able to get to your bug-out location on time.

Heatwave

Underground bunkers are also really cool and will keep you comfortable during a heatwave.

Floods and Fires

Be careful not to use an underground bunker in case of fires or floods, unless your bunker is specifically designed to handle these natural disasters.

2. Artificial Disasters

As society becomes more and more unfair, we will see more artificial disasters. To be honest, this is very scary, but don't forget that therefore you became a prepper in the first place: to banish fear by being prepared.

Nuclear War

As more countries join the nuclear arms race, some using their "bomb" as a threat to adjoining countries or even the superpowers, the possibility of a nuclear war is as real as it was in the 1980s.

During the 80s, nuclear fallout shelters for private use became quite popular, albeit controversial. Some of these shelters were factory-built, fitted out, and shipped to the site where they were buried deep in the ground and surrounded by concrete. Others were made on-site using reinforced concrete and then fitted out before covering in dirt.

Both of these options are still available today, but they are extremely expensive and the technical requirements are quite stringent to withstand a nuclear blast and radiation fallout. They require emergency power, air filtration systems, and air-tight doors. Not something that can be constructed by the keen amateur.

EMPs

Bunkers are also built to withstand electromagnetic pulses (EMPs). EMPs occur after a nuclear explosion happens, statically charging the lower atmosphere. EMPs will damage all your electronic devices, as well as electrical power grids, leaving you with no ability to contact loved ones or emergency services.

Similarly, a bunker will protect you from Coronal Mass Ejections (CMEs). These are released plasma and magnetic fields ejected from our sun. Once CMEs reach Earth, they can do damage to electrical power grids.

Long-Term Power Outages

With CMEs or EMPs, you could suddenly find yourself without electricity for weeks and even months. Our entire survival system depends on electricity and energy. Most supermarkets only stock food that lasts one or two days at most. Food will go bad and farms will start being looted as chaos ensues. As humans turn on each other, your best bet for survival is a bunker.

Pandemic

Pandemics can be natural or artificial, but, without a doubt, they are always a danger to you. We saw with the recent COVID-19 pandemic outbreak how easy it is for pathogens to spread and infect the entire Earth's population. It took just a few weeks, but with an even more powerful superbug, it can take just days. We also saw with COVID-19 how isolation helped stop the spread of superbugs. If a bunker isn't a great place to isolate, then we don't know what is.

Cyber Attack

Our entire lives are governed by the internet and our electronic devices. With widespread cyber attacks, society would crumble within the space of days, leading to social breakdown.

Social Breakdown

We have seen more and more civil unrest in recent years, as society seems to break down, albeit slowly. It takes just one civil unrest to turn into an entire societal breakdown. In fact, it takes just one event to lead to an entire social breakdown, as we saw in the lead-up to World War I.

You never know what will lead to social breakdowns, so it is best to just be prepared by having a bunker.

HOW TO BUILD A BUNKER

Before you start digging, there are a few things you must consider. First, what is it you want to protect yourself from? As we mentioned earlier, nuclear bunkers are not something you can build yourself, so let's come down a level and look at the other natural and artificial disasters that you can defend against at a reasonable cost.

1. Choose Your Location

Your location must be in a safe, secret, and private area that is within walking distance of your house. As already discussed, bunkers do not fare well when introduced to fire or water, so avoid areas near bodies of water or flammable material, like dry grass.

Don't locate your bunker close to trees or vegetation because the roots will make it difficult to dig and you don't want to cut through them, as this could make trees unstable and kill off smaller plants.

2. Develop a Blueprint

Your bunker is designed for safety, security, and comfort—not luxury. This means that you're not wasting any space on unnecessary things, but you still need space to move around comfortably.

The best way to do this is to make the best use of vertical space. Go for bunk beds rather than a king-size bed. Install wall-mounted furniture, like tables and storage units. An open-plan design allows you to combine space for sitting, eating, and preparing food. You may have separate rooms for sleeping, which can be formed using timber and plasterboard partitions, but you certainly will need to separate the toilet area.

We recommend you plan for between 5-10 square feet of space per person. This will give you some idea of the area you need for your bunker. A long, narrow design is better than a square design, as this will keep the span of the roof to a minimum.

Consider also how you will get in and out of the bunker—steps or a ladder. Ladders are not suitable for a disabled person but they take up less room.

Draw your blueprint to scale, showing the correct wall thicknesses and where all the furniture and equipment will go. There are many free software packages available that you can use if you're no good at drawing.

3. Pick the Right Bunker Material

Your bunker must support the weight of the surrounding earth and the backfill material on top. There are several materials you can use, these are the most popular:

Metal Sheeting

Profiled or corrugated metal sheeting is water-resistant and sturdy, but it must be supported on a steel frame. The roof steelwork will need vertical support as well, which might impact your floor layout.

Metal sheeting will also need insulating and lining if you don't want to see the bare metal.

Concrete

Concrete is the best material for the floor slab, where it must be laid on a sheet of thick polythene (300 microns) to prevent water rising from the ground.

Concrete can also be used for the walls and roof, but it must be reinforced with steel bars or mesh, and again, protected from water ingress.

Wooden shuttering is required to form the walls and roof, which may even be left in place on the inside to make it easier to fix things.

Bricks and Blocks

Bricks and blocks are easy to lay and cheap to source. Blocks are quicker to lay being larger than bricks, but they're not as aesthetic.

For perimeter walls, it is best to build the outer leaf using dense concrete blocks and an inner leaf of brick with a cavity between them to prevent groundwater from penetrating the inside surface.

4. Get Your Permit

Don't start any construction work until you have a permit from your local building department or zoning board. For this, you will need your blueprint and a map of where your bunker will be located.

Depending on where you live, you may also need one or more of the following: grading permit, discretionary permit, plumbing permit, and electrical permit. If you intend to have ventilation equipment installed, you will also need a permit for that.

Armed with your permits, there is one more thing you must do before you start digging, and that is to call 811. This is the utility hotline and they will tell you where the pipes and lines are in the area where you want to dig.

5. Choose the Right Excavating   Equipment

You're going to need an excavator (or mini-excavator) for this. Digging by hand is not only arduous and slow, but it is also dangerous at this kind of depth.

Set out the area of your bunker with pegs and rope using the dimensions on your blueprint. It's best to add a foot all around to allow for discrepancies in the digging.

6. Start Digging

The excavation needs to be as deep as your bunker plus around 2-3 feet for dirt cover.

Excavating is a hazardous operation and there are lots that can go wrong that can lead to injuries or even death. As a precaution, you must:

- Keep excavators and heavy equipment away from the edge of the excavation.

- Keep a ladder in the excavation at all times.

- Don't allow exhaust fumes from plant such as generators or vehicles to discharge over the excavation.

- Barrier around the excavation at the end of a day's work.

The type of soil you're digging into will inform you about the type of support you need. Cohesive soil has a high clay content, so the sides of the excavation should stay vertical while you build the walls. Granular soil contains sand and gravel, so you will have to support the sides or slope/bench them.

Sloping is done by cutting the trench wall at an angle, whereas benching is done by creating long benches that rise up the wall in steps.

7. Construct the Shelter

Start with the floor. We recommend using reinforced concrete for the floor because it is strong and forms a good base for the walls.

Once the base of your excavation is flat and free of vegetation, place a 4-inch layer of stone over the whole area and compact it. This will help drain away any groundwater and take up any ground movement. Place a 2-inch layer of sand over this so the surface is flat and free of any sharp stone.

Next, place a layer of polythene over the sand with about a foot left over at the edges, which should be turned up against the sides of the excavation.

It is quicker and cheaper to use a welded mesh reinforcement on the floor. This must be spaced 2 inches off the polythene so the concrete can get underneath it when it's poured.

If you're mixing your own concrete, a mix of 1 part cement, 2 parts sand, and 3 parts stone by volume will be strong enough.

With your base laid, you can build the shelter using the materials of your choice. You can even place a pre-fabricated shelter on the slab, or if your budget is tight, a shipping container, but this would have to be reinforced to withstand the pressure of the surrounding earth.

Remember, the walls need to be thick enough to support the roof, and the roof needs to be strong enough to support the dirt backfill. This may mean you have to incorporate steel beams and columns.

If you live in an earthquake zone, you may also need to reinforce your bunker with cross braces, movement-resisting frames, and shear walls. An engineer will advise you on this and any other structural issues you may have.

8. Acquire Key Living Equipment

Key living equipment will keep you alive while you are underground. You will need:

Ventilation/Air Filters

To provide fresh air and filter out air contaminants.

Water Filters

You will need a UV filter while living underground to destroy viruses and bacteria.

Waste Removal System

You need a way to get rid of toxic waste once you are off-grid in your bunker. This includes:

○ A "poop tube" made with a PVC pipe. These are OK for short-term use and easy to set up.

○ A composting toilet that converts waste into fertilizer that can be used for your plants. Composting toilets can get smelly in the enclosed space of your bunker.

○ A wastewater pump and lift system. This system pumps your waste from the toilet to the ground level, keeping your bunker free of waste. Hand pumps avoid the need for an electrical supply.

A Backup Generator

Although you may have connected your bunker to your domestic electricity supply, there is no guarantee that this will be available after a catastrophic event. A backup generator will provide you with electricity for lighting and ventilation for as long as you have enough fuel.

Locate the generator somewhere outside your bunker or in its own below-ground storage unit because the exhaust fumes are highly toxic.

9. Stock Up On Provisions

Stock up on food and water provisions. See Chapter Four to decide what food and drinks to store. Some preppers argue that two weeks' worth of food is enough, but this is not a good idea.

In the event of a nuclear explosion or a biological/chemical attack, you may have to sit out the aftermath for up to six months before radiation or contamination levels subside enough for you to venture out. Therefore, six months should be considered the optimum period for storage purposes.

SURVIVAL TASK

Although bunkers can be more costly than other shelters, it could be life-saving, particularly if there was a nuclear attack. Seriously consider implementing a Plan C shelter option.

Take two minutes to think about a location where you could build a bunker. Look back over this chapter and come up with a few ideas on how you could structure your bunker. If a disaster is looming, then you need to be prepared!

Key Chapter Takeaway

- In case of situations where you would have to evacuate your home, it is essential to have other shelters or safe houses prepared.

- Shelter is even more important than water and food if you want to survive in the short and long term.

- Shelter protects you from long-term exposure to the elements and the outside world, which could cause hypothermia (becoming too cold), hyperthermia (becoming too hot), and many other dangerous conditions.

- Any shelter you build should keep you dry, repelling wind and rain.

- Don't be tempted to choose either bugging out or bugging in over the other just because one method suits your specific situations better. Prepare for both!

- If bugging in, you will need to fortify your home to protect you from looters or even violent rioters.

- On your way to your bug-out shelter, you will need to construct a temporary shelter to keep you alive. Your temporary shelter must protect you from wild animals, other humans, and the elements.

- An underground bunker is optional, but highly recommended, in case of natural/manmade disaster, or in case you cannot reach your bug-out location before disaster strikes.

In the next chapter, you will learn basic first aid techniques that you could use effectively on yourself and your family should anyone become injured.

CHAPTER SEVEN:
FIRST AID

First aid is paramount to your survival during a disaster. As a prepper, you probably already know the importance of basic first aid. Yet, you might feel that you're too busy or it's not that important. Let's face it, all of us fall for that human arrogance of thinking that bad things will never happen to us: accidents only happen to other people.

Once the shit hits the fan, however, you can count on one thing: accidents will become more common. Even worse, it might be the case that emergency services are no longer functional. So, how do you and your survival party stay healthy and alive in that case? Plus, first aid is a lot more than staying alive. As a prepper, your first goal is staying alive, but you also have other goals. First aid will help you to:

1. Reduce Danger

Imagine that you are on your way to your bug-out location when a member of your survival party is bitten by an animal. They are bleeding profusely and will die within a few hours if you cannot bandage up the wound temporarily.

Also, you cannot continue your journey because you will leave a trail of blood that leaves you all in danger of both predators and other people who may want to rob you of your supplies - or worse! With first aid, you and your survival party can continue on your journey as quickly as possible without being exposed to predators, bad weather, and other humans.

2. Stay Healthy and Safe

Knowing how to take care of your basic medical needs keeps you healthy and safe from things like infections and medical complications. With first aid training comes great physical health, mental clarity, and a good immune system, all of which help you to stay healthy and alive during a disaster.

3. Prevent Your Conditions From Getting Worse

Leaving infections, wounds, and other health problems without treatment is just a gateway for your condition to get worse. This can lead to permanent disability or even death.

4. Be Confident

A great prepper is confident in their ability to survive. If not, you wouldn't prepare in the first place. You have taken the hard route of embracing the truth for what it is, so don't do things halfway. Now that you have embraced the truth, you want to have all the training you need, so that you can be confident that you will survive any scenario.

5. Increase Comfort

Nobody wants to be in pain - especially not during a disaster. A first aid kit, and first aid training, will reduce your survival party's chances of dealing with pain and suffering.

This chapter aims to inform you of basic first aid techniques that you could use effectively on yourself, your family, and anyone in your survival party, should anyone become injured. You will learn the importance of packing your own first aid kit, how many first aid kits you need, and the seven areas of first aid you need to prep for. Finally, you will understand why every good prepper has a **PERM**:

- **P**lace a first aid kit in every bag and location.

- **Enroll** in first aid class.

- **R**egularly practice emergency scenarios.

- **M**odify your first aid kit to fit your individual needs.

WHY YOU SHOULD PACK YOUR OWN KIT

Most preppers don't realize that they need to pack their own first aid kit. You can buy pre-packed first aid kits, which is highly convenient. The only problem is that they are created for everyday life. You use the tools in a first aid kit until you can either call emergency services or get to the hospital. At most, this will take you a day. This differs greatly from a first aid kit for when shit hits the fan. You don't know how long it's going to be until you can get to an emergency center or a hospital, so you must pack a heavy-duty trauma kit if you are to survive. With a heavy-duty trauma kit, you can take care of many different injuries, including serious traumatic injuries.

SEVEN AREAS OF FIRST AID FOR PREPPERS

These are the seven areas that you must pack in your first aid kit. Pack them in an easy-to-transport bag, so that you can grab the bag in case of emergencies.

1. Diarrhea

Diarrhea (watery bowel movements) can be caused by bacteria, viruses, parasites, medications, lactose intolerance, fructose intolerance, and any other digestive disorders. If left untreated, for even a few days, diarrhea can kill!

Remember that you will have to drink filtered water and possibly eat meat that you have to hunt yourself, without modern-day sanitation practices. To put it another way, diarrhea is an ever-present threat in disaster mode. Luckily, with the proper medication, you can prevent diarrhea by stocking the following:

- Activated charcoal tablets (to prevent poisoning).

- Enzyme supplement (for keeping your digestive system healthy).

- Fresh Green Black Walnut Wormwood Complex (for treating parasites).

- Heartburn relief, such as Tums or generic brands.

- Anti-diarrheal, for example, Imodium or any generic brand.

- Apple cider vinegar (to calm your stomach and indigestion and to prevent yeast infections).

- Electrolyte replenishing drinks, such as clear broth, Pedialyte (for children in your survival party), or just a teaspoon of salt mixed in apple juice.

2. Wound Treatment

Your first aid kit should be able to treat and protect against scrapes, punctures, cuts, burns, wounds, blisters, stings, bites too hot or too cold skin, and radiation burns. Care for your skin by stocking:

- Sunscreen lotions

- Soap

- Rubbing alcohol

- Neosporin/Polysporin

- Hydrogen Peroxide

- Moleskin

- Hydrocortisone anti-itch cream (for skin irritation)

- Bandages

- Burn Jel

- Blister Medic (for your feet)

- Ibuprofen (for relieving pain and swelling)

- Instant cold packs (for relieving pain and swelling)

- QuickClot

- Tweezers

- Sterile Scissors

- Splints

- Steri Strips skin closure

3. Upper Respiratory Infections

Don't let the medical-sounding name fool you. Upper respiratory infections just mean things like a cough, sore throat, and runny nose. It could also just mean things like lethargy or difficulty breathing. You will need:

- Antihistamine

- Halls Cough Drops

- Flash Light (for checking your throat in the dark)

- Thieves Oil (to prevent upper respiratory infections)

- Hydrogen Peroxide (to remove phlegm, mucus, or other secretions associated with a sore mouth)

4. Pain and Fever

Pain and fever can be caused by bacterial infections, heat, viruses, sunburn, and being exhausted, so pack:

- Mercury-free Analog Oral Thermometer

- Ibuprofen (for relieving pain, fever, and swelling)

- Chemical heat and cold packs

- Fish Mox (amoxicillin you can get over the counter without prescription)

5. Flu and Pandemic

Avoid the spread of flu, colds, bird flu, and swine flu by packing:

- Respirators (pandemic gloves)

- Nitrile Exam Gloves (stored in zip-lock bags to prevent contamination with nasty bugs)

- Pandemic Flu Kit. (Designed by Sundstrom, the Pandemic Flu Kit comes with a 99.997% absorption particle filter to filter out harmful particles like bacteria and viruses

- Infection Protection Kit (which contains eye protection, disposable thermometers, N95 respirator masks, vinyl gloves, and biohazard bags)

6. Dental Emergencies

For dental emergencies, carry:

- Hydrogen peroxide (for keeping your teeth clean)

- Hurricane Topical Anesthetic Gel

- Dental Medic. A dental first aid kit, Dental Medic, has the tools you need to treat dental pain and injury. It can serve as a replacement dental visit until you cannot get to a dentist

7. Personal Emergencies

For any other personal medical emergencies, stock:

- First aid for allergies/anaphylactic shock (Get two Epi-pens and Benadryl)

- First aid for diabetes (Store insulin in refrigerated containers and glucose tablets)

- First aid for eye care (Stock a few bottles of Visine. Make sure that the tip of the bottle does not hit another surface, or it will become infected)

This list is just a basic guide. What we recommend is that you take stock and think about what every member in your survival party truly needs. Then, you can tailor the kits to these needs.

8. What You Need To Do Now

Here is a step-by-step list of what you will need to do next to prepare.

1. Enroll in a First Aid Class. You can search for local first aid classes online to learn how to administer good first aid.

2. Practice emergency scenarios regularly. Practice emergency scenarios regularly. That way, it becomes routine for you. When an emergency occurs, sometimes it triggers our brain into freeze mode and we become paralyzed with shock. Practise beforehand to avoid being frozen in an actual emergency.

3. Evaluate your own requirements for an emergency first aid survival kit. What do you need specifically based on your needs and the needs of others in your survival party?

4. Buy a good first aid manual. Purchase two physical copies: one for home and one placed in your safety first aid kit. If you prepare more than two first aid kits, then you need a first aid manual in all of them.

You can also download a PDF first aid manual to your smartphone to use for reference in case of emergencies. It is better to download it now when you have internet service. If you wait, there might not be 4G or Wi-Fi services available when you really need them.

9. How Many First Aid Kits Do I Need?

From this chapter alone, you now realize that you need multiple first aid kits for multiple purposes and to suit the different needs of everyone in your survival party.

You will also need a first aid kit in your bug-out bag, your get-home bag, your bug-in location, and your safe location. That is a lot of first aid kits to prepare, so evaluate what you will need in each kit. You may not need a dental first aid kit in your bug-out bag, for example, if you are using it to simply head to your safe location, where you have one.

Key Chapter Takeaway

- First aid is paramount to your survival during a disaster. It helps you stay safe from danger, stay healthy and comfortable, and prevents your health conditions from getting any worse.

- You need to pack your own heavy-duty trauma kit if you are to survive when SHTF.

- Your first aid kit must be tailored to meet your specific needs.

- Pack your first aid kit in an easy-to-transport bag, so that you can grab the bag in case of emergencies.

- It is important to enroll in a first aid class and practice emergency scenarios regularly.

- Buy good first aid manuals and keep one in every location and every bag.

- Download a PDF first aid manual to keep on your phone in case of emergencies.

In the next chapter, you will learn the different ways to create an off-grid waste system so that you can become more self-reliant and more likely to survive a scenario where you are forced to cope on your own.

CHAPTER EIGHT:
CREATING AN OFF-GRID WASTE SYSTEM

As we've seen throughout this book, once the shit hits the fan, all the normal utilities that we depend on so heavily as part of our everyday lives may become a thing of the past. By now, you should understand that, although disaster takes away the feelings of safety and security we take for granted in our everyday lives, prepping gives you the confidence and peace to accept a new reality.

This chapter deals with a utility that we take for granted: waste management. Why do we take it for granted? Well, we've become accustomed to a world where waste is disposed of regularly, or kept out of sight.

But all you need to do is spend a few days in a bunker with no waste management before you realize, with panic, how and why waste management is so important for staying healthy and alive. Apart from the horrendous, you will feel sick and may quickly fall ill - not to mention all the bugs and critters that will suddenly find their way to your bunker, home, or temporary shelter.

In this chapter, we will teach you how to avoid this nightmare by building your own waste management system, specifically greywater treatment systems and blackwater treatment systems. We will also show you how to get an off-grid water supply without a well.

What's more, with the information in this chapter, you can become more self-reliant and more likely to survive a scenario where you are forced to cope on your own, without usual waste management services available, whether it be government-assisted waste management, plumbers, or others. To meet your off-grid waste and water needs, you need to follow the three Rs:

- Reuse water

- Recycle your water and waste

- Rainwater is free to collect

GREYWATER TREATMENT

Before we move on to discussing the differences between greywater and blackwater, you need to know how cities and municipalities deal with their waste. Sewage systems have a simple mechanism where interconnected pipes collect all our waste into a treatment plant. There, the waste-filled water is filtered, disinfected, and treated until it is safe to use once more.

Greywater is separated from blackwater because it contains less waste, such as dirt, food waste, human skin cells, and cleaning products. With less toxic waste, like food waste and human waste, it contains less harmful pathogens and bacteria. That means you only need minimal treatment before you can reuse it in your garden and even toilet bowls. You can connect the pipes from your washing machines, sinks, tubs, and showers to collect gray water. Once you collect greywater, you can:

1. Leach It

To leach greywater, you connect your pipes to the irrigation system in your garden. That way you can use the greywater to water your plants. The soil helps break down and treat the water before the plants, then use it. You just have to ensure that your irrigation system only waters the soil, but doesn't touch your plants.

2. Treat It

You can purchase your own professional greywater system, to treat and disinfect your greywater. This usually comes in the shape of a compact closed bucket that passes the water through many stages of filtration. Then the filtered greywater moves into your irrigation system to automatically water your garden.

3. Refill Your Toilet

Last, you can replace the top of your toilet with a special sink and tap that connects to your toilet, allowing you to wash your hands with clean water. The sink then collects that greywater so that you can use it to flush your toilet.

BLACKWATER TREATMENT

Blackwater waste, as we've mentioned, has much more pathogens and bacteria in it because it contains more waste, especially harmful waste, including urine and feces. As a result, you will have to thoroughly treat it in your off-grid system before it can be reused. Another problem with blackwater waste is that it smells terrible.

If you cannot stand bad smells, then you might think of using blackwater waste as a Plan B to greywater waste. Or, you can leave the treatment systems outside far away from your home so that you do not smell it. There are three off-grid systems available to you. They are:

1. Composting Toilets

Composting toilets collect your human waste, then mix it with natural substances, such as pine needles, coffee grounds, and wood shavings. You then leave it in a bucket or container and give it time to turn into compost. To speed up the process, you can also add it to a composter, which provides enough heat to turn it completely into compost safe enough for your garden. A lot of preppers like to use Nature's Head brand of composting toilets.

You can also create your own DIY composting toilet. This is one drawback of being a prepper. Once the government and businesses stop functioning to meet your needs, you really do have to do it yourself, even when meeting your needs involves building and using a compost toilet.

But, there are advantages to a DIY composting toilet. They might smell terrible, but they are very cheap to make and they don't require any water for flushing, so you don't have to worry about providing water for your toilet from your finite water supply.

The silver lining is that they are very easy to make. You only really need a toilet seat, a bucket, and some wood shavings. However, they can be very smelly and you don't want to end up in a situation where the bucket tips. So you can design an outdoor toilet that looks similar to a cupboard with doors.

The doors keep the smell away and leave everything contained. Also, make sure that you change the bucket regularly (every 2-3 days) and add wood shavings to the feces after every use.

We recommend that you add a urine diverter to your DIY composting toilet. Feces compost much quicker when dry, so you want to keep urine away from it. A urine diverter sounds very fancy, but it is just a funnel added to the front of the toilet bowl, on the inside, to catch your urine in a urine chamber and keep it separate from feces. The urine chamber should be emptied every 2-3 days. You have the option to then treat your urine separately or to use it as a source of nitrogen for your garden.

As a word of caution, you need very high temperatures to kill all the pathogens in blackwater compost. We advise that you purchase a composter, otherwise it can take up to two years without high temperatures to treat your compost.

2. Septic Tanks

Septic tanks can be placed underground and connected to your house through perforated pipes. They allow for oils and fats in the waste to rise to the top and for solids to sink to the bottom. Then, the wastewater by-product moves on to the second section, where it flows out through your garden irrigation system into the "leach field", i.e. your garden's soil. The soil then does the job of breaking down and filtering the water while the fats and solids remain in the tank.

With most septic systems, you need to empty them out (pumping them out) every 3 to 5 years.

A survival party with 3-4 people will need a septic tank that can hold 1,000 gallons (between 90-120 inches long and 60-80 inches wide). You will also need to lay the pipes in your leach field, so your leach field needs to measure about 4,500 square feet (about 100 feet long and 45 feet wide).

Do not install your septic system yourself. While it is possible to do so, using a professional gives you the reassurance that they have done it properly. The last thing you want during a disaster is to have your septic tank burst, with no professional to help you deal with it. Not to mention, you just simply cannot take your chances with things like human waste. If they contaminate your food and water supply, it could kill you within the space of just a few days. In this case, you do not want to take any chances!

You will also be most likely required by law to have it inspected before use. As you can imagine, failing inspections over and over again is expensive. Some states and municipalities require that your septic tank be installed by a professional. It simply is in your best interest to hire a professional from the outset.

3. Aerobic System

Aerobic systems are similar to septic tanks, except it is divided into 6 or 7 sections. The first 2-3 sections use the same anaerobic breakdown process as a septic tank. In the last sections, oxygen is pumped in to help the bacteria in the waste break it down through an aerobic process. Unlike a septic tank, you get much cleaner water that is then released into the soil.

Thanks to its added sections, septic tanks need more parts and upkeep and are more expensive. However, they are definitely worth it if you can afford one.

Before choosing what off-grid wastewater and waste management system you want to implement, check your local laws! There may be restrictions and requirements that you must abide by. If you feel that the restrictions and requirements are unlawful, then you can mount a legal challenge.

HOW TO GET AN OFF-GRID WATER SUPPLY WITHOUT A WELL

In case you don't have access to a well, collecting rainwater is the next best alternative.

Most people don't know that just one inch of rain falling on an area measuring about 1,000 square feet can yield up to 600 gallons. The Environmental Protection Agency (EPA, 2022) states that the average American home uses 300 gallons of water daily. Unfortunately, it does not rain every day.

If you were to collect all the water that fell on your roof in all of 2019, you could only collect 59,126 gallons of rainwater (Off-Grid Home, 2022a). That means you can only get half of your annual water needs from rainwater. In that case, conserving and managing your collected rainwater is paramount to survival. You will also need to:

- Reduce the amount you use. You can take a shower every two days instead of daily, for example.

- Recycle water using the greywater tips discussed in this chapter.

- Create a larger area for rain collection by using frames and tarps.

- Supplement rainwater by buying some water or finding an alternative source, like a river.

The good news is that a rainwater system has many variables. That means that you can set it up to suit your property, as well as the resources you have available. Four ways to collect rainwater are:

1. The Roof

Clean the gutters around the lower edges of your roof area or install gutters if you have none.

Install filters in the gutters and in the downpipe.

Add a first flush diverter to your downpipe to divert the first few gallons of dirty water that run off your roof.

Place a container below your downpipe to catch the water.

2. Tarp

Dig a basin-shaped hole in the ground, about a few inches deep to match the size and shape of your tarp.

Make sure the hole is lower in one corner to create a flow.

Lay your tarp into the hole, ensuring the edges curve up to prevent water from running off the edge.

Run a pipe or rigid hose from the lower corner into a container.

3. Frame

Create a large, inclined, smooth surface, such as rigid plastic sheeting, and hold it off the ground using a rigid frame. Add guttering at the lower edge to collect the rainwater into your collection container.

4. Direct Container

Place as many open containers outside as possible to collect rainwater. Empty them regularly, to prevent algae from growing and to keep mosquitoes away.

5. Rainwater Above-Ground

Store your rainwater in big above-ground storage containers. If possible, place it next to your house or on a rooftop/elevated surface. That way, minimal piping, and guttering are needed.

SURVIVAL TASK

Think about which system you think is most appropriate for you to get. How quickly could you get it fitted? How would each different element fit into your emergency plan? For example, if the plan was to move to another safe location, then would it be more effective to install an off-grid waste management system where your safe location is?

Never use light-colored containers, as the sunlight on the container will cause algae to grow. Use opaque black or green containers instead. In cold weather, wrap the heating tape around your containers and pipes to prevent your water from freezing.

Collecting rainwater is cheap because, apart from the price of containers - which are affordable - you can swap full containers for empty ones to collect more water (if you keep your storage above ground).

Key Chapter Takeaway

- Greywater is separated from blackwater because it contains less waste, such as dirt, food waste, human skin cells, and cleaning products.

- Greywater only needs minimal treatment before you can reuse it in your garden and even toilet bowls.

- Blackwater waste has much more pathogens and bacteria in it because it contains more harmful waste, including urine and feces.

- Before choosing what off-grid wastewater and waste management system you want to implement, check your local laws! There may be restrictions as well as requirements that you must abide by.

- In case you don't have access to a well, collecting rainwater is the next best off-grid alternative.

In the next chapter, you will learn the importance of being prepared for any scenario, particularly when it comes to protecting yourself and your loved ones.

CHAPTER NINE:
PROTECTING YOURSELVES

This chapter aims to highlight the importance of being prepared for any scenario, particularly for protecting yourself and your loved ones. You will learn how to know your enemy, use lethal and non-lethal tools, as well as DIY weapons, and use defensive tactics under fire.

SIX THINGS NOT TO DO

Here are six things a good prepper never does in order to stay safe:

1. Bragging About Your Supply

The first thing any seasoned prepper will tell you is to never share with others that you are a prepper. In times of desperation, anyone can turn against you. Protect yourself by keeping your prepper status secret and sharing only with people who are in your survival party.

2. Relying on One Form of Defense

Remember that a good prepper always has a Plan A, Plan B, and Plan C. So practice and prepare to use more than one form of defense, from hand-to-hand combat to guns, to non-lethal weapons.

3. Only Stockpiling Guns and Ammo

Lethal weapons are not needed in every scenario. Sometimes you can deescalate a situation with non-lethal weapons, so it is best to stockpile other forms of weapons apart from guns and ammo.

4. Not Bugging Out

No matter how much you try to defend or protect your house, you may need to leave if it is compromised by enemies. Always have a packed bug-out bag ready to leave at a moment's notice.

5. Shooting on Sight

Not everyone approaching you or your shelter is an enemy. Someone may just be approaching for help or out of curiosity. Resist the urge to shoot on sight, as it can just escalate a situation badly. Always have the mentality that you are protecting yourself, not attacking others.

6. Not Defending Your Home Well Enough

As we've seen in chapter 6, there are severe consequences for not defending your home well enough, so don't make this mistake.

KNOWING YOUR ENEMY

Knowing your enemy and defending yourself from your enemy is pivotal for survival. But who is your enemy? That's the worrying part about shit hitting the fan: anyone can be your enemy, be it looters, hungry beggars, or thirsty neighbors who find out you have water. Other potential enemies include rioters and organized gangs. The great news is that, if you take the precautions listed in **chapter 6**, as well as those listed in this chapter, you can protect yourself if the time comes.

Non-Lethal Tools

Here are some non-lethal tools you can keep on hand for self-defense.

1. Bear Spray

Bear spray is just pepper spray for bears. If sprayed near a bear, the bear will most likely stay away from you and even leave because they could not breathe.

2. Stun Gun and Taser

Check your state and local laws to ensure that owning a stun gun and taser is legal. If it is then purchase both. Stun guns require direct contact (i.e. being physically close to the assailant), while tasers work even a few feet from your assailant.

3. Pepper Spray

Pepper spray is one of the best non-lethal weapons out there. Once you use it on an assailant, they cannot breathe and it burns their eyes severely. This gives you enough time to escape. You also don't need to be close to a person to use pepper spray. You can be a few feet away from them.

4. Kubotan

Learn how to use the Kubotan in self-defense. While it requires you to be close to the assailant, you can purchase one with a pepper spray that enables you to stay far from your assailant. It allows you to incapacitate them with the pepper spray before you then approach them and use your Kubotan on them.

Lethal Tools

If a person appears as though they intend to harm you, then you are well within your right to use a lethal tool against them.

1. Firearms in Restrictive States

If you live in a restrictive state, you can still carry a pump shotgun or a lever-action rifle in a mid-weight cartridge.

2. Firearms in Open States

In open states, carry semi-automatic pistols and rifles. They are the most reliable guns against someone who wants to harm you.

3. DIY Weapons

In case you don't have the above weapons on you, you can make your own DIY weapons, like:

- Spears

- Blowguns

- Primitive Club Tools

- Balloon Slingshots

- Stun Grenades

DEFENSIVE TACTICS WHEN UNDER FIRE

Here are some defensive tactics you can use when under fire:

- Force Dispersal

- Fanning Out

- Positioning along a diagonal line

- Protective tactics for your family

- Weaponry

- Codes/safety systems

SURVIVAL TASK

Now that you have everything to defend yourself, you can complete the next task. This is a very important task as part of the preparation required for catastrophe, so don't skip it.

First, recap this chapter. Reflect on why defense is important, but also think about what defense is right for you.

If you are not comfortable shooting people, then it may be better to concentrate on non-lethal weapons, for example.

Next, do a stock check. What weapons do you already have? What weapons do you still need? Things like kitchen knives can come in very handy, so don't forget them. Using the template below, create a list of the weapons you currently have and take stock of what you need to do to get really prepared.

Firearms	Other Lethal Weapons	Non-Lethal Weapons

Key Chapter Takeaway

- Knowing your enemy and defending yourself from your enemy is pivotal for survival.

- Worryingly, when shit hits the fan, anyone can be your enemy.

- If a person seems as though they want to harm you, then you are well within your right to use a lethal tool against them.

- Not everyone who approaches you is an enemy. Try not to use lethal weapons unless you are sure they want to harm you.

In the next chapter, you will learn how to create an emergency plan, whether this is just for yourself or for your entire survival party.

CHAPTER TEN:
CREATING AN EMERGENCY PLAN

Now that you have all the tools you need to create an emergency plan—whether for you, your family, or anyone else in your survival party—you must spend time carefully creating your emergency plan to meet the needs of everyone in your party. This plan could, ultimately, be the difference between life and death in a life-threatening catastrophe.

As you create your plan, always keep in mind that you need to *P.O.P!*

- *P*lan, plan, plan!

- *O*rganize your plans!

- *Practice* drills!

Don't worry if you don't know how to create or organize your emergency plan. That is why we are here.

THE GOALS FOR YOUR EMERGENCY PLAN

There are four major goals that your emergency plan aims to achieve:

1. Staying Safe

A prepper is firstly concerned with survival. Well, how do you survive? By staying safe. Your plan must consider safety at every step. How do you drink safe, clean water when you're bugging out? Do you fortify your house against intruders? What do you pack in your first aid kit to meet the health needs of everyone in your survival party? Remember that your emergency plan must be tailored to meet the needs of everyone in your survival party.

2. Limiting Loss

There is no point storing a year's supply of food only to find that it has been damaged or infested with pests.

Prepping costs money, so you want to limit your losses. Otherwise, you are throwing money away.

3. Reuniting Quickly

Your emergency plan will have details of where to meet in case your survival party is separated.

4. Resuming Normal Life ASAP

The life of a prepper is difficult and requires a lot of resilience. You will want to prepare how to transition back into normal life ASAP.

8 STEPS FOR CREATING AN EMERGENCY PLAN

Here are eight easy steps for creating an emergency plan:

1. Plan Now

As has been discussed in this book, disaster can strike at any moment. Trust us! You will regret not planning now if disaster strikes tomorrow.

2. Assess What Will Happen

What could realistically happen based on where you live? You don't expect a person who lives in Australia to prep for a snowstorm. So, what are the likely scenarios to occur in your area, whether political or societal upheaval or natural or manmade disasters?

3. Communicate With Family and Friends

There is no point in making a survival plan for your friends and family and not informing them of it. If the goal is for them to survive, then they must study your plan as well as have input in its creation.

4. Make a Shelter and Secure Your Home

As has been discussed in previous chapters, you will need to include in your plan details for making a shelter and securing your home. If there are any shelters you can make now or any way you can secure your home now, then you will also need to do that.

5. Know How Long Supplies Will Last

Your plan should account for how long supplies will last. Food is precious in an emergency and you can't just eat as you would. Rationing and planning will go a long way in keeping you alive.

6. Have Books/Resources on Survival Skills

As we said in the introduction, the prepping community is still relatively new. There is so much to learn, with information constantly being released. It is in your best interest to keep up with the community by reading books, visiting websites, and watching videos made by other preppers.

7. Keep Your Plan Flexible

You should have several unique plans for different scenarios. Ideally, you will have at least one plan for bugging out and one plan for bugging in. Your plan should be flexible enough that you can still follow it should detail change. If you plan to survive on your bean rations for three months and it runs out after the second month, you should be able to find another protein source in your food stockpile to last you the next month.

8. Keep Your Information Safe

In today's world, when you need your identification documents to do practically everything, you want to ensure that you keep your identity documents safe. The best way to do this is to scan them onto an online drive. This way, you always have electronic copies, in case you lose physical copies.

Second, always leave them stored securely in your bug-out bag in waterproof bags. That way, if you ever need to leave home, you will have your identity documents with you. You may need them to cross a border, for example.

Everyone in your survival party must also keep a small booklet with the contact information of everyone else. In case of separation, this booklet might be the one thing to reunite you. This contact information should also be stored in the online drive, along with identity documents.

In addition, everyone's bug-out bag must have physical copies of the emergency plan. It gives everyone time to study and familiarize themselves with it. The plan must also contain details of emergency meeting places for everyone in your survival party. You must decide on a primary and secondary meeting place, in case of separation. In your plan, there must also be details of your out-of-area meeting place.

ORGANIZING YOUR PLAN

Most preppers like to use binders to organize their plan. You can then place these binders in important locations, such as your car, office, your children's locker at school, and your bug-out bags.

If you have kids, encourage them to read the plan and become familiar with worst-case scenarios so that, if an emergency strikes, they won't panic. Instead, they could go straight into action.

Your binder should contain:

- Contact information of everyone in your survival party. In addition, include the contact information of other people that you know, for example, grandparents, neighbors, teachers, and anyone and everyone who may be of help during a disaster

- Include all allergy and medical information in binders

- Response plans to likely scenarios in your area

- Responsibilities of everyone in your survival party. If disaster strikes, who puts out the containers to collect rainwater? Who unplugs all devices in the house? Create a list of necessary tasks

- Make physical copies of personal identification documents such as passports and driver's licenses

- Food storage information, including expiry date and how much food you have

- Details (and maps) of emergency meeting places

Last, practice drills with everyone in your survival party. This is a great way to prevent anyone from freezing out of shock and, ultimately, not surviving as a result

SURVIVAL TASK

This book has given you the knowledge you need to now write an in-depth plan for any catastrophe. Your best tool for survival is this plan. Once you've thought every detail through, you will be completely prepared to adapt to multiple situations that could happen. When things go wrong, this will be your most valuable asset.

Key Chapter Takeaway

- Your emergency plan could, ultimately, be the difference between life and death in a life-threatening catastrophe.

- Organize your plan in binders, then place them in strategic locations, such as your car, office, or children's school lockers.

In the next chapter, you will do a final check-in. Now that you have read the book, you know exactly what to do when things go wrong.

Chapter Eleven:
A Final Check-In

This chapter is your final preparation phase. Once you have completed this check-in exercise, you will know exactly what you need to do to become more prepared and live off the grid, should the need for it arise.

Check-in Exercise

Now you have finished the book, let's first explore where you are right now in your prepping for the worst-case scenario journey.

Below, rate yourself on a scale of 1- 5 on how accurate the statements are for you. A score of 1 means "not accurate," and a score of 5 means "very accurate." After you have rated yourself according to the statements, add the total of your scores, then read "What Your Score Really Means" to determine the outcome of your results.

Check-in Statement

Check-in Statement	Self-Rating
I am completely sure that I can live off-grid.	

I have a detailed idea of what it takes to be self-sufficient.	
My bug-out bag contains everything I need to survive for 3 days.	
I know where I will source water and how to purify it.	
I have stored food for emergencies and am now food self-sufficient.	
I have decided whether it is best for me to bug-in bug-out. I know how to fortify my home for bugging in and how to create my own bunker or shelter for bugging out.	
I have a basic knowledge of first aid to treat either myself or my family.	
I know how to create a basic off-grid waste system.	

I know how to keep myself safe from enemies during disasters.	
I have an emergency plan for any disaster scenario that could happen right now.	
TOTAL SCORE:	

WHAT YOUR SCORE REALLY MEANS

Score: 10-15

You are not prepared for a disaster and will struggle to keep yourself and your family safe during an emergency.

Did you skip any chapters? Maybe you should have another read...

Score: 16 - 30

You have a basic understanding of what it means to be a prepper, but you should review your strategies and make changes to enhance your preparedness.

Well done! This is definitely good progress. Draw up a plan of how you can even better your knowledge. Review any chapters you were a little unsure about and make sure your plan is perfect.

Score: 31+

You are almost ready for survival during a disaster! Review your plans to ensure they are ready to go.

Great job. You have put yourself in a powerful position for any catastrophe that may occur.

Don't be discouraged if you haven't scored well. Reread the sections you scored low on to fully understand the information and get back on track to being prepared.

If you scored well in this check-in exercise, then congratulations are in order! You are now fully prepared for survival in the case of a disaster!

FINAL WORDS

This has been a long journey, but you finally made it: you have all the information that you need to survive when shit hits the fan. From experience, we know how empowered you must feel knowing that you can survive no matter what happens. This is not a feeling that most people get to experience. You certainly deserve to enjoy your accomplishment because it took a lot of work and guts to get through this book. Congratulations!

As you go on to implement all the survival guides that we have brought you, we hope you keep in mind that you are doing this for your survival and the survival of your loved ones. All the hard work will pay off!

You may find that, as you begin to store your food and prepare for water shortages, family and friends will become more interested and invested in prepping too. You are simply a trendsetter who will go on to save the lives of many.

The great news is that you now have all this knowledge to share with others around you who may become interested in prepping, from how to pack a bug-out bag, to how much water to store for survival; how to source water, purify water, and how to store food properly to survive for months and even years!

You even know how to cook without power and how to build your oven as a long-term cooking solution. As if that's not enough, you now know how to build temporary shelters and your underground bunker. You know how to pack a survival first aid kit and how to secure your home against intruders.

Last, you know how to create off-grid waste systems and how to protect yourself from anyone or any animal that may want to attack you. You have a detailed emergency plan and you know the importance of sticking to it. Even better, you have the tools that you need in case you need to deviate from your emergency plan.

You are now prepared to face the unknown and deal with what could be a major catastrophe, so remember to keep this guide handy for hints and tips when SHTF.

We leave you one last piece of advice: disaster can strike at any moment, so always stay prepared. In the words of the great Carl Sagan, "Extinction is the rule. Survival is the exception."

DID YOU ENJOY THE BOOK? WE'D LOVE TO HEAR YOUR THOUGHTS!

Thank you for purchasing & reading our book! We do have a favor to ask from you, and that's if you can leave a review on our Amazon page!

As a small, independent publishing company with a tiny marketing budget, reviews are our livelihood on this platform. Even if it's just a sentence or two, it would make all the difference and would be very much appreciated.

If you already have, we'd like to thank you so much for leaving the review!

If you haven't yet, you can simply write your review here on our page through one of these links or scan the QR Codes.

If you're from the US, you can leave a review by clicking this link or scanning the code:

https://amazon.com/review/create-review?&asin=1804210154

If you're from the UK, you can leave a review by clicking this link or scanning the code:

https://amazon.co.uk/review/create-review?&asin=1804210154

We pour our heart and soul into our books, and reviews like yours help us spread our message and get our work into the hands of more people.

We appreciate you, and we just want to say thank you.

Sincerely,

Small Footprint Press

REFERENCES

Ames, H., & Bell, A. M. (2020, December 11). **Can you sleep with a concussion? What happens and when to seek help.** www.medicalnewstoday.com. https://www.medicalnewstoday.com/articles/can-you-sleep-with-a-concussion?c=613291398967

Angie. (2014, February 28). Chinese medicine first aid - Part one: Nosebleeds, conjunctivitis & burns. Angie Savva Acupuncture. https://www.angiesavva.com/blog/chinese-medicine-first-aid-part-one-nosebleeds-conjunctivitis-burns

Are you prepared for a medical emergency? (2018, January 1). Harvard Health. https://www.health.harvard.edu/staying-healthy/are-you-prepared-for-a-medical-emergency

Basic first aid procedures - Quick tips #207 - Grainger KnowHow. (2016, January 7). https://www.grainger.com/know-how/health/medical-and-first-aid/first-aid/kh-safety-basic-first-aid-procedures-207-qt

Beatty, K. (n.d.). Natural first aid kit. Simple Tens; Simple Tens-Karla Beatty. *Retrieved June 28, 2021, from* https://www.simpletens.com/natural-first-aid-kit.html

Borke, J., Zieve, D., Conaway, B., & ADAM Medical Editorial Team. (2019). Recognizing medical emergencies: MedlinePlus Medical Encyclopedia. *Medlineplus.gov.* *https://medlineplus.gov/ency/article/001927.htm*

Caraway: Uses, side effects, dose, health benefits, precautions & warnings. *(n.d.). EMedicineHealth; WebMD Inc. Retrieved July 3, 2021, from* https://www.emedicinehealth.com/caraway/vitamins-supplements.htm

Chappell, S., & Stevens, C. *(2019, February 21).* A beginner's guide to making herbal salves and lotions. *Healthline.* *https://www.healthline.com/health/diy-herbal-salves*

Cheong, T. (2019). **How to survive an asthma attack if you're caught without your inhaler.** Healthxchange.sg. **https://www.healthxchange.sg/asthma/complications-management/survive-asthma-without-inhaler**

Cirino, E., & Carter, A. (2019, August 28). What is a Tincture? Herbal Recipes, Uses, Benefits, and Precautions. *Healthline.* https://www.healthline.com/health/what-is-a-tincture#summary

Dave. (2014, July 10). **Homemade: Plantain anti-itch salve and lotion bars.** Happy Acres Blog. **https://happyacres.blog/2014/07/09/homemade-plantain-anti-itch-salve-and-lotion-bars/**

Emergency Responders: Tips for taking care of yourself. *(2018).* *CDC.gov.* https://emergency.cdc.gov/coping/responders.asp

Emily. (2018, March 14). **Natural, homemade postpartum wipes and cooling spray. naturally free**.

https://www.naturallyfreelife.com/natural-diy-tucks-wipes-and-postpartum-cooling-spray/

Engineer, R. (2018, August 8). **Be prepared: 10 Common medical Emergencies & How to Deal With Them.** The Better India. https://www.thebetterindia.com/155315/first-aid-medical-emergencies-news/

Eske, J., & Chauvoustie, C. T. (2020, December 8). **Too much hydrogen peroxide in ear: Risks, safety, treatment, and more.** www.medicalnewstoday.com. https://www.medicalnewstoday.com/articles/too-much-hydrogen-peroxide-in-ear#risks

First aid basics and DRSABCD. (2012). Vic.gov.au. https://www.betterhealth.vic.gov.au/health/conditions andtreatments/first-aid-basics-and-drsabcd

First-aid kits: Stock supplies that can save lives. (2018). Mayo Clinic; https://www.mayoclinic.org/first-aid/first-aid-kits/basics/art-20056673

Fisher, S. (2020, October 23). **Clean naturally with these best DIY disinfectants.** The Spruce. https://www.thespruce.com/best-diy-disinfectants-4799867

Fletcher, J., & Cobb, C. (2019, June 7). **9 Home remedies for burns and scalds.** www.medicalnewstoday.com. https://www.medicalnewstoday.com/articles/319768#how-severe-is-the-burn

388

Fletcher, J., & Whitworth, G. (2020, January 9). **How to stop heart palpitations: 7 Home remedies and tips.** Www.medicalnewstoday.com. **https://www.medicalnewstoday.com/articles/321541?c =1339616399082#home-remedies**

Frostbite: Causes, symptoms, stages, treatment & prevention. *(n.d.). Cleveland Clinic; Cleveland Clinic. Retrieved July 1, 2021, from https://my.clevelandclinic.org/health/diseases/15439-frostbite*

Get Licensed UK. (2021). Basic first aid training UK (Updated 2021). *Www.youtube.com; Get Licensed UK. https://www.youtube.com/watch?v=ErxKDbH-iI*

Gillen, D. (2013, August 23). The wonders of witch hazel - A must have for your first aid preparations. *PreparednessMama.* https://preparednessmama.com/wonders-of-witch-hazel/

Glenn. (2015, January 29). **Top 11 natural/alternative medicine emergency first aid items. emergency food NZ. https://freezedriedemergencyfood.co.nz/top-11-natural-medicine-emergency-first-aid-items/**

GUIDE TO LOCAL PRODUCTION: WHO-RECOMMENDED HANDRUB FORMULATIONS. *(n.d.).* https://www.who.int/gpsc/5may/Guide_to_Local_Production.pdf?ua=1

Hammett, E. (2019). The latest advice on burns. BDJ Team, 6(10), 16–18. https://doi.org/10.1038/s41407-019-0186-3

Healthline Editorial Team, & Luo, E. K. (2015, September 26). **Concussion: Symptoms, diagnosis, and treatments. Healthline.** https://www.healthline.com/health/concussion?c=160 0259764957#longterm-effects

Healthwise Staff, Bladh, W. H., Thompson, E. G., Husney, A., & Romito, K. (n.d.). Chest problems | Michigan Medicine. www.uofmhealth.org. Retrieved July 2, 2021, from https://www.uofmhealth.org/health-library/cstpn#hw86215

Healthwise Staff, Blahd, W. H., Husney, A., & Romito, K. (n.d.). Head Injury, Age 4 and Older | Michigan Medicine. www.uofmhealth.org. Retrieved July 1, 2021, from https://www.uofmhealth.org/health-library/hdinj#hw93594

Healthwise Staff, Blahd, W. H., Husney, A., & Romito, K. (2020a, February 26). Dealing with emergencies | Michigan Medicine. www.uofmhealth.org. https://www.uofmhealth.org/health-library/emerg#hw154557

Healthwise Staff, Blahd, W. H., Husney, A., & Romito, K. (2020b, February 26). Shock | Michigan Medicine. www.uofmhealth.org. https://www.uofmhealth.org/health-library/shock#tp16305

Healthwise Staff, Blahd, W. H., Romito, K., & Husney, A. (2018). Poisoning: Home treatment. Mayo Clinic; https://www.uofmhealth.org/health-library/poins#tw9579

Healthwise Staff, Blahd, W. H., Romito, K., Husney, A., Thompson, E. G., O' Connor, H. M., & Gabica, M. J. (2020, February 26). Burns and electric shock | Michigan Medicine. *www.uofmhealth.org.* *https://www.uofmhealth.org/health-library/burns#hw109096*

Healthwise Staff, Romito, K., & Husney, A. (n.d.). How to stop bleeding. *www.uofmhealth.org. Retrieved July 1, 2021, from* *https://www.uofmhealth.org/health-library/zm6160#zm6160-sec*

Healthwise Staff, Romito, K., Husney, A., & Gabica, M. J. (2018, August 8). Splinting. *The Better India.* *https://www.uofmhealth.org/health-library/sid41216#sid41216-sec*

Healthwise Staff, Thompson, E. G., Husney, A., Gabica, J., & Ryan, L. (2020, September 23). Taking a pulse (Heart Rate) | Michigan Medicine. *Www.uofmhealth.org.* *https://www.uofmhealth.org/health-library/hw201445#hw201445-sec*

Heidi. (2020, September 14). **DIY herb-infused witch hazel.** Blog.mountainroseherbs.com. **https://blog.mountainroseherbs.com/herb-infused-witch-hazel**

Here are your survival kit essentials. (2019). Mayo Clinic; **https://www.mayoclinic.org/first-aid/emergency-essentials/basics/art-20134335**

Higuera, V., & Han, S. (2017, November 13). **What to do when someone is having a stroke.** Healthline.

391

https://www.healthline.com/health/stroke-treatment-and-timing/dos-and-donts

Hill, A., & Butler, N. (2019, December 6). Caraway: Nutrients, benefits, and uses. *Healthline.* *https://www.healthline.com/nutrition/caraway#bottom-line*

How to make homemade hand sanitizer. (n.d.). Franciscan Missionaries of Our Lady Health System. https://fmolhs.org/coronavirus/coronavirus-blogs/how-to-make-homemade-hand-sanitizer

Iftikhar, N., & Morrison, W. (2018, November 1). Severed finger: First aid, surgery, and recovery. *Healthline.* *https://www.healthline.com/health/severed-finger*

Iftikhar, N., & Wilson, D. R. (2019, July 23). Benefits of fennel seeds for gas, plus how to use them. *Healthline.* *https://www.healthline.com/health/fennel-seeds-for-gas*

Irene. (2019, August 13). How to make herb-infused oils for culinary & body care use. *Blog.mountainroseherbs.com.* https://blog.mountainroseherbs.com/making-herbal-oils

John Hopkins Medicine. (2019). **Acupuncture.** John Hopkins Medicine. https://www.hopkinsmedicine.org/health/wellness-and-prevention/acupuncture

Kate. (2014, June 17). **Non-Toxic DIY waterproof sunscreen.** Real Food RN. https://realfoodrn.com/diy-waterproof-sunscreen-thats-good-skin/

Krebs-Holm, L. (2019, December 20). **Ginger: Health benefits, nutrition, & how to take it.** EMediHealth. **https://www.emedihealth.com/nutrition/ginger-benefits-risk**

Laycock, R. (2021, February 18). Doomsday preppers: How many are preparing for the end? | Finder.com (C. Choi, Ed.). *Finder.com; Finder.com/Hive Empire PTY Ltd.* https://www.finder.com/doomsday-prepper-statistics

Leestma, B. (2016, April 18). **Natural disinfecting with vinegar and hydrogen peroxide.** The Make Your Own Zone. **https://www.themakeyourownzone.com/homemade-disinfecting-spray-ideas/**

Lindberg, S., & Weatherspoon, D. (2020, July 6). **How to Make Your Own Hand Sanitizer.** Healthline. **https://www.healthline.com/health/how-to-make-hand-sanitizer#how-to-use**

Lubbers, W. (2017). Emergency Procedures (C. K. Stone & R. L. Humphries, Eds.). Access medicine; McGraw-Hill Education. *https://accessmedicine.mhmedical.com/content.aspx?booki d=2172§ionid=165057582*

Mahboubi, M. (2018). Caraway as important medicinal plants in management of diseases. *Natural Products and Bioprospecting, 9(1), 1–11.* https://doi.org/10.1007/s13659-018-0190-x

Malaria. (n.d.). Www.who.int. Retrieved June 28, 2021, from *https://www.who.int/health-topics/malaria#tab=tab_3*

Marcin, A., & Wilson, D. R. (2017, March 27). **How to stop heart palpitations: 6 Home remedies and more.** Healthline. https://www.healthline.com/health/how-to-stop-heart-palpitations

Marengo, K., & Snyder, C. (2021, May 14). What Is an herbal tonic? Benefits, weight loss, and efficacy. *Healthline.* https://www.healthline.com/nutrition/herbal-tonic

Marr, K. (2016, December 4). **Homemade hand sanitizer spray (kid-friendly).** Live Simply. https://livesimply.me/homemade-hand-sanitizer-spray-kid-friendly/

Mayo Clinic. (2017a). **Concussion - diagnosis and treatment - mayo clinic.** Mayoclinic.org; https://www.mayoclinic.org/diseases-conditions/concussion/diagnosis-treatment/drc-20355600

Mayo Clinic. (2017b). **Concussion - Symptoms and causes.** Mayo Clinic; https://www.mayoclinic.org/diseases-conditions/concussion/symptoms-causes/syc-20355594

Mayo Clinic Staff. (n.d.-a). **First aid for food poisoning.** Mayo Clinic. Retrieved July 1, 2021, from https://www.mayoclinic.org/first-aid/first-aid-food-borne-illness/basics/art-20056689

Mayo Clinic Staff. (n.d.-b). Foreign object in the ear: First aid. *Mayo Clinic. Retrieved July 1, 2021, from*

https://www.mayoclinic.org/first-aid/first-aid/basics/art-20056709

Mayo Clinic Staff. (n.d.-c). Foreign object in the nose: First aid. *Mayo Clinic. Retrieved July 1, 2021, from https://www.mayoclinic.org/first-aid/first-aid/basics/art-20056610*

Mayo Clinic Staff. (n.d.-d). **Human bites: First aid.** Mayo Clinic. Retrieved July 1, 2021, from **https://www.mayoclinic.org/first-aid/first-aid-human-bites/basics/art-20056633**

Mayo Clinic Staff. (2017a). **Choking: First aid.** Mayo Clinic; **https://www.mayoclinic.org/first-aid/first-aid-choking/basics/art-20056637**

Mayo Clinic Staff. (2017b). **Nosebleeds: First aid.** Mayo Clinic; **https://www.mayoclinic.org/first-aid/first-aid-nosebleeds/basics/art-20056683**

Mayo Clinic Staff. (2018a). **Electrical shock: First aid.** Mayo Clinic; **https://www.mayoclinic.org/first-aid/first-aid-electrical-shock/basics/art-20056695**

Mayo Clinic Staff. (2018b). **Fainting: First aid.** Mayo Clinic; **https://www.mayoclinic.org/first-aid/first-aid-fainting/basics/art-20056606**

Mayo Clinic Staff. (2018c). **First aid for anaphylaxis.** Mayo Clinic; **https://www.mayoclinic.org/first-aid/first-aid-anaphylaxis/basics/art-20056608**

Mayo Clinic Staff. (2018d). **Head trauma: First aid.** Mayo Clinic; https://www.mayoclinic.org/first-aid/first-aid-head-trauma/basics/art-20056626

Mayo Clinic Staff. (2018e). **Headache: First aid.** Mayo Clinic; https://www.mayoclinic.org/first-aid/first-aid-headache/basics/art-20056639

Mayo Clinic Staff. (2018f). **Poisoning: First aid.** Mayo Clinic; https://www.mayoclinic.org/first-aid/first-aid-poisoning/basics/art-20056657

Mayo Clinic Staff. (2018g). **Spider bites: First aid.** Mayo Clinic; https://www.mayoclinic.org/first-aid/first-aid-spider-bites/basics/art-20056618

Mayo Clinic Staff. (2018h). **Sprain: First aid.** Mayo Clinic; https://www.mayoclinic.org/first-aid/first-aid-sprain/basics/art-20056622

Mayo Clinic Staff. (2019a). **Fever: First aid.** Mayo Clinic; https://www.mayoclinic.org/first-aid/first-aid-fever/basics/art-20056685

Mayo Clinic Staff. (2019b). **Hypothermia: First aid.** Mayo Clinic; https://www.mayoclinic.org/first-aid/first-aid-hypothermia/basics/art-20056624

Mayo Clinic Staff. (2019c). **Snakebites: First aid.** Mayo Clinic; https://www.mayoclinic.org/first-aid/first-aid-snake-bites/basics/art-20056681

Mayo Clinic Staff. (2019d). **Which treatment is best for your headaches?** Mayo Clinic;

https://www.mayoclinic.org/diseases-conditions/chronic-daily-headaches/in-depth/headaches/art-20047375

Mayo Clinic Staff. (2019e, July 24). **Gastroenteritis: First aid.** Mayo Clinic. https://www.mayoclinic.org/first-aid/first-aid-gastroenteritis/basics/art-20056595

Mayo Clinic Staff. (2020a, April 1). **Heatstroke: First aid.** Mayo Clinic; https://www.mayoclinic.org/first-aid-heatstroke/basics/art-20056655

Mayo Clinic Staff. (2020b, May 30). **Sunburn: First aid.** Mayo Clinic. https://www.mayoclinic.org/first-aid/first-aid-sunburn/basics/art-20056643

McDermott, A. (2018, June 4). First Aid for Stroke. *Healthline; Healthline Media.* *https://www.healthline.com/health/stroke/stroke-first-aid*

McDermott, A., & Sullivan, D. (2017, April 3). **Home remedies to stop bleeding.** Healthline. https://www.healthline.com/health/home-remedies-to-stop-bleeding#witch-hazel

Medical emergency preparation. (n.d.). www.parentgiving.com. Retrieved June 28, 2021, from https://www.parentgiving.com/elder-care/prepare-for-a-medical-emergency/

Mental Health Commission of Canada. (n.d.). Mental health first aid COVID-19 self-care & resilience guide. *Mental Health Commission of Canada. Retrieved July 3, 2021, from*

https://www.mhfa.ca/sites/default/files/mhfa_self-care-resilience-guide.pdf

Merissa. (2014, March 10). **The best burn salve recipe.** Little House Living. **https://www.littlehouseliving.com/best-burn-salve.html#_a5y_p=1511158**

Mrs Happy Homemaker, C. (2012, November 1). **Healing Boo-Boo Salve - aka Homemade natural neosporin.** Mrs Happy Homemaker. **https://www.mrshappyhomemaker.com/healing-boo-boo-salve-a-k-a-homemade-natural-neosporin/**

NHS Choices. (2019). **Asthma attacks - Asthma.** Nhs. **https://www.nhs.uk/conditions/asthma/asthma-attack/**

Nicholson, D. (2020, April 22). **Improvised first aid afloat.** Practical Sailor. **https://www.practical-sailor.com/blog/improvised-first-aid-afloat**

Options for first aid if no first aid kit is available. *(n.d.). Redcross.org.uk; British Red Cross Society. Retrieved June 28, 2021, from* *https://www.redcross.org.uk/first-aid/no-first-aid-kit-no-problem*

Peppermint Oil. *(n.d.).* *NCCIH.* *https://www.nccih.nih.gov/health/peppermint-oil*

Petre, A. (2018, December 19). What Is Vegetable Glycerin? Uses, Benefits and Side Effects. *Healthline; Healthline Media.* *https://www.healthline.com/nutrition/vegetable-glycerin*

Piazza, G. M., American College Of Emergency Physicians, & Dk Publishing, Inc. (2014). First aid manual : the step-by-step guide for everyone. *Dk Publishing.*

Quarantine at home - coping tips | betterhealth.vic.gov.au. (n.d.). www.betterhealth.vic.gov.au. https://www.betterhealth.vic.gov.au/health/Conditions AndTreatments/quarantine-at-home-coping-tips

Raychel. (2017, June 13). **How to make herbal tinctures.** Blog.mountainroseherbs.com. https://blog.mountainroseherbs.com/guide-tinctures-extracts

Raypole, C., & Moawad, H. (2019, June 14). Concussions and sleep: A dangerous mix? *Healthline.* *https://www.healthline.com/health/concussion-and-sleep*

Rescue Remedy drops and spray - Original Rescue Remedy. *(n.d.). Information & Sales - the Original Bach Flower Remedies; Bachflower.com. Retrieved June 28, 2021, from* *http://www.bachflower.com/rescue-remedy-information/*

Santos-Longhurst, A., & Marcin, J. (2018, July 9). What to Do When You or Someone You Know May Have Breathed in Too Much Smoke. *Healthline; Healthline Media.* *https://www.healthline.com/health/smoke-inhalation*

Schauf, C. (2019, March 12). 10 Basic first aid training tips & procedures for any emergency. *Uncharted Supply Company; Uncharted Supply Company.* *https://unchartedsupplyco.com/blogs/news/basic-first-aid*

Seladi-Schulman, J. (2019, April 25). About peppermint oil uses and benefits. *Healthline; Healthline Media.* *https://www.healthline.com/health/benefits-of-peppermint-oil*

SkylerRyser. (2019, February 7). **Three C's of an emergency & three P's of first aid.** Idaho Medical Academy. **https://www.idahomedicalacademy.com/the-three-cs-of-an-emergency-and-the-three-ps-of-first-aid/**

Stewart, J. (2015, March 23). **Hydrogen peroxide + vinegar = A disinfecting duo?** Cleaning Business Today. **https://cleaningbusinesstoday.com/blog/hydrogen-peroxide-vinegar-a-disinfecting-duo/**

Stroke treatment. *(2019). Centers for Disease Control and Prevention. https://www.cdc.gov/stroke/treatments.htm*

The World's Most Natural First Aid Kit. (2013, January 4).   Redbook. **https://www.redbookmag.com/body/health-fitness/advice/a14796/acupressure-points-chart/**

Thompson, E. G., Gabica, M. J., Romito, K., Husney, A., & Zorowitz, R. D. (2020, March 4). Stroke | Michigan Medicine. *www.uofmhealth.org.* *https://www.uofmhealth.org/health-library/hw224638#hw224684*

Traditional Chinese Medicine could make "Health for One" true.   *(n.d.).* https://www.who.int/intellectualproperty/studies/Jia.pdf

Traveler's   first   aid   kit. (n.d.). www.emergencyphysicians.org. Retrieved June 28, 2021, from **https://www.emergencyphysicians.org/article/health—safety-tips/travelers-first-aid-kit**

Vukovich, L. (n.d.). **Make your own natural first-aid kit.** Motherearthliving.com. Retrieved June 30, 2021, from **https://content.motherearthliving.com/health-and-wellness/make-your-own-natural-first-aid-kit/**

Watson, K., & Wilson, D. R. (2019, July 10). Homemade sunscreens: Can you make one that is safe and effective? *Healthline.* https://www.healthline.com/health/homemade-sunscreen

WHO, I. (1997). Management of poisoning - A handbook for health care workers: Part 1 - General information on poison and poisoning: Chapter 5 - First aid: First aid for poisoning. *Helid.digicollection.org.* http://helid.digicollection.org/en/d/Js13469e/4.5.3.html

You can Stop bleeding in less than 60 seconds! | Go Beyond Organic. (2012, May 4). www.gobeyondorganic.com. **http://www.gobeyondorganic.com/you-can-stop-bleeding-in-less-than-60-seconds**

Alexa, R. (2021, May 2). Bugging In: How To Fortify Your Home For SHTF. Tactical. https://www.tactical.com/fortify-your-home-shtf/.

Alexa, R. (2018, April 18). Should You Bug In Or Bug Out When SHTF? Tactical. https://www.tactical.com/should-you-bug-in-or-bug-out/.

Berkey Filters. (2022). Berkey Filter Test Results. Berkey Filters. https://www.berkeyfilters.com/pages/filtration-specifications.

BigRentz Inc. (2020, July 20). How To Build An Underground Bunker In 9 Steps. Big Rentz. https://www.bigrentz.com/blog/how-to-build-underground-bunker.

Blair, C. (2022). How Long Can Water Be Stored Before it Goes Bad? EZ Prepping. https://ezprepping.com/how-long-can-water-be-stored-before-it-goes-bad/.

Bryant, R. (2014). Defensive Tactics When Under Fire. The Prepper Journal. https://theprepperjournal.com/2014/08/29/defensive-tactics-fire/amp/.

Bug-Out Bag Builder. (2022). Bug-Out Bag Builder Checklist. https://www.bugoutbagbuilder.com/sites/default/files/images/Bug-Out-Bag-Builder-Checklist.pdf.

Burton-Hughes, L. (2017, May 17). What Are 'The Big 8' Food Allergies? High Speed Training. https://www.highspeedtraining.co.uk/hub/common-food-intolerances-allergies/.

402

Collier, E. (2019, August 26). What Are The Four Types Of Food Contamination? High Speed Training. https://www.highspeedtraining.co.uk/hub/four-types-contamination/.

Conroy, J.O. (2020, April 30). We Mocked Preppers And Survivalists - Until The Pandemic Hit. The Guardian. https://www.theguardian.com/global/2020/apr/30/preppers-survivalists-disasters-lessons.

Denzer, K. (2022). Build Your Own Wood-Fired Earth Oven. Mother Earth News. https://www.motherearthnews.com/diy/build-your-own-wood-fired-earth-oven-zmaz02onzgoe/.

Emergency First Response Corp. (2022). 5 Reasons Why Basic First Aid Knowledge Is Essential. Emergency First Response Corp. https://www.emergencyfirstresponse.com/5-reasons-why-basic-first-aid-knowledge-is-essential/.

Engel Fires. (2018, October 26). The Benefits Of Wood Fired Cooking. Engel Fires. https://www.engelfires.co.nz/blog/benefits-wood-fired-cooking.

Gamble, E. (2020, August 21). 5 Reasons Why You Need A Bug-Out Bag. Eric Gamble. https://www.ericgamble.com/5-reasons-why-you-need-a-bug-out-bag/.

Global Water Group. (2022). Difference Between Blackwater And Greywater. Global Water Group.

https://www.globalwatergroup.com.au/our-blog/difference-between-blackwater-and-greywater.

Happy Preppers. (2022). Bleach Storage Tips For Beginners. Happy Preppers. https://www.happypreppers.com/bleach.html.

Happy Preppers. (2022). First Aid Kits. Happy Preppers. https://www.happypreppers.com/First-aid.html.

Happy Preppers. (2022). Prepper Medicine Cabinet. Happy Preppers.https://www.happypreppers.com/medicine-cabinet.html.

Happy Preppers. (2022). Water Survival Guide. Happy Preppers. https://www.happypreppers.com/water.html.

Jones, K. (2022). Be Part Of The Solution: 14 Compelling Reasons To Be A Prepper. The Provident Prepper. https://theprovidentprepper.org/be-part-of-the-solution-14-compelling-reasons-to-be-a-prepper/.

Kimble, B. (2022). 9 Celebrity Preppers Ready For Anything. Ready Wise. https://readywise.com/blogs/readywise-blog/9-celebrity-preppers-ready-for-anything.

Kylene. (2022). Be Part Of The Solution: 14 Compelling Reasons To Be A Prepper. The Provident Prepper. https://theprovidentprepper.org/be-part-of-the-solution-14-compelling-reasons-to-be-a-prepper/.

Kylene. (2022). Emergency Water: 17 Potential Sources. The Provident Prepper.

https://theprovidentprepper.org/emergency-water-17-potential-sources/

Kylene. (2022). Ingenious Places to Store Your Emergency Food Supply. The Provident Prepper. https://theprovidentprepper.org/ingenious-places-to-store-your-emergency-food-supply/.

Kylene. (2022). Steps To Build A Successful Family Emergency Plan. The Provident Prepper. https://theprovidentprepper.org/steps-to-build-a-successful-family-emergency-plan/.

Kylene. (2022). Top 10 Foods To Hoard For "The End of The World As We Know It". The Provident Prepper. https://theprovidentprepper.org/top-10-foods-to-hoard-for-the-end-of-the-world-as-we-know-it/.

Lussier, M. (2018, May 30). 5 Reasons To Grow Your Own Food. University Of New Hampshire. https://www.unh.edu/healthyunh/blog/nutrition/2018/05/5-reasons-grow-your-own-food.

Mel C. (2021, June 4). The Get Home Bag Vs. The bug-out Bag Vs. The Go Bag. Tactical. https://www.tactical.com/get-home-bag-vs-bug-out-bag-vs-go-bag/.

Merriam-Webster. (2022). Bug-Out Bag. Merriam-Webster. https://www.merriam-webster.com/dictionary/bug-out%20bag#:~:text=Definition%20of%20bug%2Dout%20bag,rapid%20evacuation%20%3A%20go%20bag%20When%20%E2%80%A6.

Mr BOBB. (2016, April 11). How To Build A $20 Budget Friendly Bug Out Bag. Bug-Out Bag Builder. https://www.bugoutbagbuilder.com/blog/best-20-budget-bug-out-bag-build.

Mr BOBB. (2019, August 26). Survival Self-Defense Weapons For Prepper's. Bug-Out Bag Builder. https://www.bugoutbagbuilder.com/blog/survival-self-defense-weapons-preppers.

Off-Grid Home. (2022). The Complete Guide To Off-Grid Wastewater Management. Off-Grid Home. https://off-grid-home.com/guide-to-off-grid-wastewater/.

Off-Grid Home. (2022). How To Get An Off-Grid Water Supply Without A Well. Off-Grid Home. https://off-grid-home.com/how-to-get-an-off-grid-water-supply/.

OHare, M. (2019, June 14). Spending Time In Nature Boosts Health, Study Finds. CNN. https://edition.cnn.com/travel/article/nature-health-benefits/index.html.

Preissman, D. (2017, June 28). How To Choose The Ultimate Bug Out Location. Tactical. https://www.tactical.com/how-to-choose-the-ultimate-bug-out-location/.

Preissman, D. (2017, June 28). What's A Bug Out Location? Tactical. https://www.tactical.com/how-to-choose-the-ultimate-bug-out-location/.

Preparedness Advice. (2020, November 26). Preppers Food Storage 101: An Ultimate Guide. Preparedness Advice. https://preparednessadvice.com/prepper-food-storage/.

Primed Preppers. (2022). Prepper Water Storage And Filtration - The Ultimate Guide. Primed Preppers. https://primedpreppers.com/prepper-water-storage-filtration/.

Rich, M. (2015, November 15). What You Really Need In Your SHTF First Aid Kit. Ask A Prepper. https://www.askaprepper.com/what-you-really-need-in-your-shtf-first-aid-kit/.

Schuaf, C. (2022, March 2). Bug-Out Bag Essentials Checklist. Uncharted Supply. https://unchartedsupplyco.com/blogs/news/bug-out-bag-checklist.

SHTFDad. (2022). 10 Reasons To Build An Underground Bunker. SHTFDad. https://www.shtfdad.com/10-reasons-to-build-an-underground-bunker/.

Sullivan, D.F. (2022). 16 Surprising Benefits Of Prepping. Survival Sullivan. https://www.survivalsullivan.com/16-surprising-benefits-of-prepping/.

Sullivan, D.F. (2022). 7 Kick Ass DIY Weapons For Your Survival. Survival Sullivan. https://www.survivalsullivan.com/7-kick-ass-diy-weapons-for-your-survival/.

Sullivan, D.F. (2022). Bug-Out Shelters. Survival Sullivan. https://www.survivalsullivan.com/bug-out-shelters/.

Sullivan, D.F. (2022). Why Shelter Is Important. Survival Sullivan. https://www.survivalsullivan.com/why-shelter-is-important/.

Survivalist 101. (2022). Emergency Water Storage: How Much Water To Store For Prepping? Survivalist 101. https://survivalist101.com/tutorials/preppers-guide-prepping-for-beginners/emergency-water-storage-how-much-water-to-store-for-prepping/.

Survivalist 101. (2022). How To Cook Food Without Power. Survivalist 101. https://survivalist101.com/tutorials/preppers-guide-prepping-for-beginners/how-to-cook-food-without-power/.

The Bug-Out Bag Guide. (2022). How To Make A Bug-Out Plan. The Bug-Out Bag Guide. https://www.thebugoutbagguide.com/how-to-make-a-bug-out-plan/.

The Prepared Way. (2019, August 19). Home Security For Preppers – Protecting Your Home And Family After SHTF. https://thepreparedway.com/home-security-for-preppers-protecting-your-home-and-family-after-shtf/.

The Prepper Journal. (2022). WROL – Protecting Your Family When The Bad Guys Come Down Your Street – Pt. 1. The Prepper Journal. https://theprepperjournal.com/2013/08/29/without-rule-of-law-protecting-your-family-when-the-bad-guys-come-pt-1/amp/.

The Prepping Guide. (2022). Prepping Basics: How To Start Prepping in 2021. The Prepping Guide. https://thepreppingguide.com/prepping-basics/.

The Provident Prepper. (2022). Emergency Cooking – Recommended Products. The Provident Prepper. https://theprovidentprepper.org/recommended-products/emergency-cooking-recommended-products/.

The Provident Prepper. (2022). SHTF Plan: How to Create Your Survival and Emergency Plans. The Provident Prepper. https://thepreppingguide.com/shtf-plan/.

The Smart Survivalist. (2022). Off Grid Septic System And Sanitation: The How-To Guide. The Smart Survivalist. https://www.thesmartsurvivalist.com/off-grid-septic-system-and-sanitation-the-how-to-guide/.

UK Preppers Guide. (2017, September 26). Safety First Aid For Preppers. UK Preppers Guide. https://www.ukpreppersguide.co.uk/safety-first-aid-for-preppers/.

Urban, A. (2022). The Beginner's Guide To Emergency Food Storage. Urban Survival Site. https://urbansurvivalsite.com/beginners-guide-to-emergency-food-storage/.

Urban Survival Network. (2022). 10 Common Prepping Mistakes Every Survivalist Should Avoid. Urban Survival Network. https://www.urbansurvivalnetwork.com/10-common-prepping-mistakes-every-survivalist-should-avoid/.

Vukovic, D. (2022, March 21). 22 Ways To Cook Without Electricity When The Grid Fails. Primal Survivor. https://www.primalsurvivor.net/ways-cook-without-electricity/.

Weston, J. (2021, April 15). 20 Items To Kick Start Your Long Term Food Storage Plan. Backdoor Survival. https://www.backdoorsurvival.com/20-items-to-kick-start-your-food-storage-plan/.

Alexa, R. (2021, May 2). Bugging In: How To Fortify Your Home For SHTF. Tactical. https://www.tactical.com/fortify-your-home-shtf/.

Alexa, R. (2018, April 18). Should You Bug In Or Bug Out When SHTF? Tactical. https://www.tactical.com/should-you-bug-in-or-bug-out/.

Berkey Filters. (2022). Berkey Filter Test Results. Berkey Filters. https://www.berkeyfilters.com/pages/filtration-specifications.

BigRentz Inc. (2020, July 20). How To Build An Underground Bunker In 9 Steps. Big Rentz.

https://www.bigrentz.com/blog/how-to-build-underground-bunker.

Blair, C. (2022). How Long Can Water Be Stored Before it Goes Bad? EZ Prepping. https://ezprepping.com/how-long-can-water-be-stored-before-it-goes-bad/.

Bryant, R. (2014). Defensive Tactics When Under Fire. The Prepper Journal. https://theprepperjournal.com/2014/08/29/defensive-tactics-fire/amp/.

Bug-Out Bag Builder. (2022). Bug-Out Bag Builder Checklist. https://www.bugoutbagbuilder.com/sites/default/files/images/Bug-Out-Bag-Builder-Checklist.pdf.

Burton-Hughes, L. (2017, May 17). What Are 'The Big 8' Food Allergies? High Speed Training. https://www.highspeedtraining.co.uk/hub/common-food-intolerances-allergies/.

Collier, E. (2019, August 26). What Are The Four Types Of Food Contamination? High Speed Training. https://www.highspeedtraining.co.uk/hub/four-types-contamination/.

Conroy, J.O. (2020, April 30). We Mocked Preppers And Survivalists - Until The Pandemic Hit. The Guardian. https://www.theguardian.com/global/2020/apr/30/preppers-survivalists-disasters-lessons.

Denzer, K. (2022). Build Your Own Wood-Fired Earth Oven. Mother Earth News. https://www.motherearthnews.com/diy/build-your-own-wood-fired-earth-oven-zmaz02onzgoe/.

Emergency First Response Corp. (2022). 5 Reasons Why Basic First Aid Knowledge Is Essential. Emergency First Response Corp. https://www.emergencyfirstresponse.com/5-reasons-why-basic-first-aid-knowledge-is-essential/.

Engel Fires. (2018, October 26). The Benefits Of Wood Fired Cooking. Engel Fires. https://www.engelfires.co.nz/blog/benefits-wood-fired-cooking.

Gamble, E. (2020, August 21). 5 Reasons Why You Need A Bug-Out Bag. Eric Gamble. https://www.ericgamble.com/5-reasons-why-you-need-a-bug-out-bag/.

Global Water Group. (2022). Difference Between Blackwater And Greywater. Global Water Group. https://www.globalwatergroup.com.au/our-blog/difference-between-blackwater-and-greywater.

Happy Preppers. (2022). Bleach Storage Tips For Beginners. Happy Preppers. https://www.happypreppers.com/bleach.html.

Happy Preppers. (2022). First Aid Kits. Happy Preppers. https://www.happypreppers.com/First-aid.html.

Happy Preppers. (2022). Prepper Medicine Cabinet. Happy Preppers.https://www.happypreppers.com/medicine-cabinet.html.

Happy Preppers. (2022). Water Survival Guide. Happy Preppers. https://www.happypreppers.com/water.html.

Jones, K. (2022). Be Part Of The Solution: 14 Compelling Reasons To Be A Prepper. The Provident Prepper. https://theprovidentprepper.org/be-part-of-the-solution-14-compelling-reasons-to-be-a-prepper/.

Kimble, B. (2022). 9 Celebrity Preppers Ready For Anything. Ready Wise. https://readywise.com/blogs/readywise-blog/9-celebrity-preppers-ready-for-anything.

Kylene. (2022). Be Part Of The Solution: 14 Compelling Reasons To Be A Prepper. The Provident Prepper. https://theprovidentprepper.org/be-part-of-the-solution-14-compelling-reasons-to-be-a-prepper/.

Kylene. (2022). Emergency Water: 17 Potential Sources. The Provident Prepper. https://theprovidentprepper.org/emergency-water-17-potential-sources/

Kylene. (2022). Ingenious Places to Store Your Emergency Food Supply. The Provident Prepper. https://theprovidentprepper.org/ingenious-places-to-store-your-emergency-food-supply/.

Kylene. (2022). Steps To Build A Successful Family Emergency Plan. The Provident Prepper. https://theprovidentprepper.org/steps-to-build-a-successful-family-emergency-plan/.

Kylene. (2022). Top 10 Foods To Hoard For "The End of The World As We Know It". The Provident Prepper. https://theprovidentprepper.org/top-10-foods-to-hoard-for-the-end-of-the-world-as-we-know-it/.

Lussier, M. (2018, May 30). 5 Reasons To Grow Your Own Food. University Of New Hampshire. https://www.unh.edu/healthyunh/blog/nutrition/2018/05/5-reasons-grow-your-own-food.

Mel C. (2021, June 4). The Get Home Bag Vs. The bug-out Bag Vs. The Go Bag. Tactical. https://www.tactical.com/get-home-bag-vs-bug-out-bag-vs-go-bag/.

Merriam-Webster. (2022). Bug-Out Bag. Merriam-Webster. https://www.merriam-webster.com/dictionary/bug-out%20bag#:~:text=Definition%20of%20bug%2Dout%20bag,rapid%20evacuation%20%3A%20go%20bag%20When%20%E2%80%A6.

Mr BOBB. (2016, April 11). How To Build A $20 Budget Friendly Bug Out Bag. Bug-Out Bag Builder. https://www.bugoutbagbuilder.com/blog/best-20-budget-bug-out-bag-build.

Mr BOBB. (2019, August 26). Survival Self-Defense Weapons For Prepper's. Bug-Out Bag Builder.

https://www.bugoutbagbuilder.com/blog/survival-self-defense-weapons-preppers.

Off-Grid Home. (2022). The Complete Guide To Off-Grid Wastewater Management. Off-Grid Home. https://off-grid-home.com/guide-to-off-grid-wastewater/.

Off-Grid Home. (2022). How To Get An Off-Grid Water Supply Without A Well. Off-Grid Home. https://off-grid-home.com/how-to-get-an-off-grid-water-supply/.

OHare, M. (2019, June 14). Spending Time In Nature Boosts Health, Study Finds. CNN. https://edition.cnn.com/travel/article/nature-health-benefits/index.html.

Preissman, D. (2017, June 28). How To Choose The Ultimate Bug Out Location. Tactical. https://www.tactical.com/how-to-choose-the-ultimate-bug-out-location/.

Preissman, D. (2017, June 28). What's A Bug Out Location? Tactical. https://www.tactical.com/how-to-choose-the-ultimate-bug-out-location/.

Preparedness Advice. (2020, November 26). Preppers Food Storage 101: An Ultimate Guide. Preparedness Advice. https://preparednessadvice.com/prepper-food-storage/.

Primed Preppers. (2022). Prepper Water Storage And Filtration - The Ultimate Guide. Primed Preppers. https://primedpreppers.com/prepper-water-storage-filtration/.

Rich, M. (2015, November 15). What You Really Need In Your SHTF First Aid Kit. Ask A Prepper. https://www.askaprepper.com/what-you-really-need-in-your-shtf-first-aid-kit/.

Schuaf, C. (2022, March 2). Bug-Out Bag Essentials Checklist. Uncharted Supply. https://unchartedsupplyco.com/blogs/news/bug-out-bag-checklist.

SHTFDad. (2022). 10 Reasons To Build An Underground Bunker. SHTFDad. https://www.shtfdad.com/10-reasons-to-build-an-underground-bunker/.

Sullivan, D.F. (2022). 16 Surprising Benefits Of Prepping. Survival Sullivan. https://www.survivalsullivan.com/16-surprising-benefits-of-prepping/.

Sullivan, D.F. (2022). 7 Kick Ass DIY Weapons For Your Survival. Survival Sullivan. https://www.survivalsullivan.com/7-kick-ass-diy-weapons-for-your-survival/.

Sullivan, D.F. (2022). Bug-Out Shelters. Survival Sullivan. https://www.survivalsullivan.com/bug-out-shelters/.

Sullivan, D.F. (2022). Why Shelter Is Important. Survival Sullivan. https://www.survivalsullivan.com/why-shelter-is-important/.

Survivalist 101. (2022). Emergency Water Storage: How Much Water To Store For Prepping? Survivalist 101. https://survivalist101.com/tutorials/preppers-guide-prepping-for-beginners/emergency-water-storage-how-much-water-to-store-for-prepping/.

Survivalist 101. (2022). How To Cook Food Without Power. Survivalist 101. https://survivalist101.com/tutorials/preppers-guide-prepping-for-beginners/how-to-cook-food-without-power/.

The Bug-Out Bag Guide. (2022). How To Make A Bug-Out Plan. The Bug-Out Bag Guide. https://www.thebugoutbagguide.com/how-to-make-a-bug-out-plan/.

The Prepared Way. (2019, August 19). Home Security For Preppers—Protecting Your Home And Family After SHTF. https://thepreparedway.com/home-security-for-preppers-protecting-your-home-and-family-after-shtf/.

The Prepper Journal. (2022). WROL—Protecting Your Family When The Bad Guys Come Down Your Street—Pt. 1. The Prepper Journal. https://theprepperjournal.com/2013/08/29/without-rule-of-law-protecting-your-family-when-the-bad-guys-come-pt-1/amp/.

The Prepping Guide. (2022). Prepping Basics: How To Start Prepping in 2021. The Prepping Guide. https://thepreppingguide.com/prepping-basics/.

The Provident Prepper. (2022). Emergency Cooking—Recommended Products. The Provident Prepper. https://theprovidentprepper.org/recommended-products/emergency-cooking-recommended-products/.

The Provident Prepper. (2022). SHTF Plan: How to Create Your Survival and Emergency Plans. The Provident Prepper. https://theproppingguide.com/shtf-plan/.

The Smart Survivalist. (2022). Off Grid Septic System And Sanitation: The How-To Guide. The Smart Survivalist. https://www.thesmartsurvivalist.com/off-grid-septic-system-and-sanitation-the-how-to-guide/.

UK Preppers Guide. (2017, September 26). Safety First Aid For Preppers. UK Preppers Guide. https://www.ukpreppersguide.co.uk/safety-first-aid-for-preppers/.

Urban, A. (2022). The Beginner's Guide To Emergency Food Storage. Urban Survival Site. https://urbansurvivalsite.com/beginners-guide-to-emergency-food-storage/.

Urban Survival Network. (2022). 10 Common Prepping Mistakes Every Survivalist Should Avoid. Urban Survival Network. https://www.urbansurvivalnetwork.com/10-common-prepping-mistakes-every-survivalist-should-avoid/.

Vukovic, D. (2022, March 21). 22 Ways To Cook Without Electricity When The Grid Fails. Primal Survivor. https://www.primalsurvivor.net/ways-cook-without-electricity/.

Weston, J. (2021, April 15). 20 Items To Kick Start Your Long Term Food Storage Plan. Backdoor Survival.

https://www.backdoorsurvival.com/20-items-to-kick-start-your-food-storage-plan/.

www.ingramcontent.com/pod-product-compliance
Lightning Source LLC
Chambersburg PA
CBHW060755100426
42813CB00004B/822